I know and respect the author although I am not comfortable with, and even disagree with, some of the thoughts he expresses in this book. But I think it is well worth reading by patients and healthcare practitioners. Minds need to be opened and patients cared for in a mindful manner so their experience and not just their diagnosis is treated. We truly need to integrate medical care, as well as explore and evaluate all the modalities that may help the people we care for and about. This book can help us move in the direction of mindful, integrated medical care for cancer and all diseases. We must remember that constructive criticism can polish our mirror. Let us read, explore and accept each other's views and in the process cure more diseases.

—BERNIE SIEGEL, M.D.
AUTHOR, *LOVE, MEDICINE AND MIRACLES*
PRESCRIPTION FOR LIVING

Dr. Contreras holds the keys to adding years to your life and life to your years. He knows that wholeness through body, mind and spirit comes from our hope in Jesus Christ, our love of God and by following the prescription of healing found in the Bible. Dr. Contreras is on a leading edge of oncology and offers health and healing to those who would hear his words.

—DR. ROBERT A. SCHULLER
CRYSTAL CATHEDRAL MINISTRIES
HOST OF *POSSIBILITY LIVING,* A DAILY RADIO HEALTH EDUCATION
PROGRAM DESIGNED TO INSPIRE PEOPLE TO MAKE POSITIVE PHYSICAL,
MENTAL AND SPIRITUAL LIFESTYLE CHANGES

The Hope of Living Cancer Free

FRANCISCO CONTRERAS, M.D.

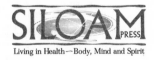

Living in Health—Body, Mind and Spirit

THE HOPE OF LIVING CANCER FREE by Francisco Contreras, M.D.
Published by Siloam Press
A part of Strang Communications
600 Rinehart Road
Lake Mary, Florida 32746
www.creationhouse.com

Unless otherwise noted, all Scripture quotations are from the King James Version of the Bible.

Scripture quotations marked NIV are from the Holy Bible, New International Version. Copyright © 1973, 1978, 1984, International Bible Society. Used by permission.

Scripture quotations marked NKJV are from the New King James Version of the Bible. Copyright © 1979, 1980, 1982 by Thomas Nelson, Inc., publishers. Used by permission.

Library of Congress Catalog Card Number: 99-75005
International Standard Book Number: 0-88419-655-0

This book is not intended to take the place of medical advice and treatment from your personal physician. Readers are advised to consult their own doctor or other qualified health professional regarding the treatment of their medical problems. Neither the publisher nor the author takes any responsibility for any possible consequences from any treatment, action or application of medicine, supplement, herb or preparation to any person reading or following the information in this book.

In order to protect the privacy of people involved, certain stories recorded in this book are composite illustrations from the histories of several individuals. Names and places have been changed, as appropriate.

0 1 2 3 4 5 6 BVG 8 7 6 5 4 3 2
Printed in the United States of America

"If God said I had a chance to reverse my cancer today,
I would say, 'Just give me one more day with cancer!'"
—John C. Riley

To John "Jack" Riley: He selflessly used his personal
battle with cancer to lead the fight for a cure and serve
others. His unshakable spirit inspired millions.

Acknowledgments

When I think about reading, the word compulsion fills my mind. I don't read just because I have to keep up with the ever-increasing medical literature. I don't read just because I love reading; it's just that I *must* read.

When I think about writing, *overwhelming* doesn't begin to describe the task at hand. This book is in your hands today because of the efforts, rather incredible efforts, of several dedicated and committed minds.

The love my father (Dr. Ernesto Contreras, Sr.) has for the patients and his immense knowledge of the art of medicine were the inspiration for this book. I wish I had the ability to weave the words into a work of art that would depict the awesome respect I have for him and the honor it is for me to share with you his invaluable medical and spiritual contributions.

The encouragement of Daniel Kennedy (Contreras) was the key that ignited the conception of this message. His tireless work and writing abilities contributed immensely in the generation of the manuscript, and his organizational genius and attention to detail were paramount for the completion of the book.

Researching and gathering the scientific, as well as the philosophical, materials to support the facts stated and the recommendations offered was a titanic task. Luisa Ruiz single-handedly accomplished it. Her selfless and relentless work has been the most powerful force behind my commitment to write.

For the medical aspects of the book, I was privileged to rely on the wise contributions from two friends and teachers of good medicine: Mario A. Soto, M.D., and Juan F. Lagos, M.D.—one an oncologist and the other an internist, both excellent doctors of bodies and souls. I also want to thank Patch Adams, M.D., and Bernie Siegel, M.D., for their commentaries and their message to patients in need in this book.

The indefatigable work of Christina Williams, my editor, is the reason why all my words make any sense to you. Her insight, sensitivity and awareness gave form and meaning to an otherwise unorganized, tremendous amount of information. She provided the cohesive, tasteful spice that makes a book palatable. I am deeply indebted to her.

I would like to thank Stephen Strang and David Welday III for having the vision of helping individuals improve their health through literature, and Rick Nash and Peg de Alminana for helping to develop and edit this book. I would also like to thank Connie Gamb, Mike Janiczek, Tammy Nelson and the entire Siloam Press team for their hard work and diligence.

The incredible support of my wife, Rosy, has me stunned. "A virtuous women, who can find?" I wish I could take the credit, but I thank God for finding her just for me. I pray God will grant me the time and energy to repay all the time that work has taken me away from her beauty and that of my five children.

But it is for my heroes that I wrote this book: Jack Riley, Laura Red, Dee Simmons, Sarah Sackett, Ruanne Crawford, Don Factor and so many other patients who have enriched my life in ways unimaginable. To them my heart and life give thanks.

Contents

Foreword

I KNOW WE have a world panic about cancer. But the worst cancer is being alive and not enjoying it, not feeling gratitude, not loving, not living. It is not the dying of death that is really a big deal; it is the dying in life that is bad. In my mind death in life is what most adults are living. To go around thinking, "Life is a struggle, life is terrible and then you die"—that's the worst cancer. Being in this miracle of life and throwing it away—that's much worse.

That is why a lot of people who get the cancer diagnosis are thankful because it wakes them up to life. It happens all the time. Cancer is so surreal; it becomes a blessing because it births the love of life. People begin to appreciate the simple and wonderful things in life like flowers and a glass of lemonade.

The hope with cancer is not whether we are going to get rid of it. Eventually this fabulous machine is going to break down, and each one of us is going to die of something. We are never going to end death. I think the big panic with getting cancer is that we are not living anyway. We want to have a little more life so we may experience the living that we have been hoping for in the future, when, in fact, anyone can it have today.

We all know cancer patients whose cancer is never more than a nuisance. Even if it eventually kills them, they enjoy life while they are alive.

If you love your life and live it in absolute fullness, then even if you get cancer, you will have lived while you were alive. That makes it all worthwhile, whether a cure comes or not.

And we need to address the environmental causes of cancer: not only the physical environmental pollution, but the emotional pollution. I don't think we know the power negative emotions have in the forming of cancer. Negative emotions that are held onto—lack of forgiveness, hostility, depression, anxiety, loneliness and lack of love that is felt all over the world—these have negative power.

Dr. Contreras's father (Dr. Ernesto Contreras, Sr.) has tried pioneering a cure. I'm sure over time, though, the things he discovered have humbled him. Anyone in complementary care knows there are new cancer ideas, therapies and cures coming out all the time from all over the world. I don't know that any one of them is ever going to resolve even 50 percent of cancer. Whoever says, "I have a cure for cancer"...well, I'm going to start thinking he is lying.

We have done some good things with childhood leukemia and other kinds of cancer. Yet we spend a huge amount of money on cancer research and almost none on love research, on how to put love back into our society. I don't know that we can prevent diseases, but we can at least live while we are living.

Almost no one is living. In my estimation, less than 90 percent of our population lives. By "lives," I mean wakes up full of vitality for life, goes to bed full of vitality of life and during the course of the day enjoys the world—the non-physical world, the physical world, the community—and ends the day saying, "I lived the today."

That is for the rich, the poor, the person with cancer, the person without, the educated, the uneducated—it is in the domain of anyone of any culture to choose this moment to say, "Thank You, thank You, God, for our lives. Thank You for music. Thank you, mother and father, for being alive. Thank you, my friend."

—PATCH ADAMS, M.D.
FOUNDER OF THE GESUNDHEIT! INSTITUTE

Dr. Adams's story was documented in the 1998 movie *Patch Adams*, starring Robin Williams. It depicted Patch's life and his struggle with conventional medical thinking. Today, Patch travels to war-torn countries to treat patients, especially children, with love, medicine and laughter.

Introduction

CANCER HAS BEEN more devastating than virtually any other plague, war or natural disaster. To put it into perspective, roughly fifty-six thousand American soldiers perished in the Vietnam War over an eleven-year period. If the war had continued for one hundred ten years, projected deaths would have reached five hundred sixty thousand. Imagine how our nation would have felt if our government had continued sending troops to war for more than a century.

Yet in America, close to five hundred sixty thousand people die from cancer in a single year—each and every year.[1] In a century's time, projected American deaths from cancer could reach fifty-six million. A tragedy.

According to the American Cancer Society, cancer will strike one out of every three people—one out of two men.[2] It is nearly impossible to find a family unaffected by this disease. The fear of cancer is much greater than the fear of any other disease. Heart disease and car accidents tend to take one's life quickly with minimal suffering. Not so with cancer, in which death can be painfully slow and cruel.

At the same time, patients dread the treatment options for

cancer. After a few rounds of chemotherapy, radiation or surgery, many patients tell their doctors that they would rather take their chances with the cancer than continue to suffer the negative side effects of the treatment.

In all this fear and suffering, a light is shining. A message of hope is emerging. Dr. Francisco Contreras, a surgical oncologist (a cancer doctor who specializes in surgery), has been empowering people to take control over cancer. He is on a mission to help people improve the quality of their physical, mental and spiritual lives. Dr. Contreras is accomplishing his mission by taking the unknowns out of the equation for cancer victims and by clearing away the confusion for those who hope to prevent cancer from striking.

Dr. Francisco Contreras was trained in conventional cancer treatments in the world-renowned First University Hospital in Vienna, Austria. Upon completion of his specialty, he returned to Mexico to work with his father, Dr. Ernesto Contreras, Sr., at their Oasis of Hope Hospital. Excited to share with his father the latest advances in cancer therapy, Francisco quickly discovered that wisdom did not come from a text book. His father, Ernesto, had been treating patients since 1939—some seventy thousand of them. Francisco found that even in hopeless cases in which patients did not respond to conventional therapy, his father was able to help the patient improve. That made Francisco a dedicated student of his father.

Dr. Ernesto Contreras, Sr., taught Francisco that when treating a patient, he should not focus on the disease, as traditional medical schools teach. Instead, the priorities are the patient's needs and his or her participation in the healing process. Each person has a body, soul and spirit, and disease can be rooted in any or all of these three realms. Ernesto taught Francisco how to design therapies that would minister to the whole person and provide resources necessary for the body to heal itself. The Contreras treatment emphasis is on the quality of the patient's life—how well he or she is doing—not the eradication of the disease at all cost.

One of the lessons Francisco learned involved a diagnostic tool called a *colonoscope*. His father called him into his office one day and inquired, "Son, I have noticed that you are ordering a colonoscopy for virtually every patient. What is that all about?"

Francisco responded enthusiastically, "We have this new instrument—a miniature camera that can be inserted into a patient so we can see everything inside the colon. It is just wonderful."

"Have you ever had a colonoscopy?"

"No."

Ernesto took out his prescription pad and ordered a colonoscopy for Francisco. Ever since Francisco had that up-close-and-personal experience with a colonoscope, very few patients at Oasis of Hope have been prescribed a colonoscopy.

This is a prime example of the Contreras' treatment philosophy, which is based on two fundamental concepts:

1. Do no harm; offer only therapies that can help the patient without sacrificing his quality of life.

2. Only recommend a therapy that you would take yourself if you had the disease. A colonoscopy is not harmful, but if it is not going to help improve the patient's condition, why order the examination?

Dr. Francisco Contreras has been leading Oasis of Hope, a top oncology center, for more than fifteen years. Oasis of Hope has been a magnet, drawing to it the most advanced conventional and alternative therapies from all around the world. Through his hospital and clinical research organization, Dr.

Contreras has identified therapies that are effective and compassionate, and he has dedicated his life to sharing this information with patients and other doctors. His experience of treating thousands of patients and researching hundreds of cancer therapies has revealed to him that the ultimate cure for cancer is *prevention.*

Through mass media, Dr. Francisco Contreras has stepped onto the world stage to reach people with important information on how to adopt a low-risk lifestyle. Although he offers no "silver bullet" and promises no cure or immunity to cancer, he imparts information, and such knowledge is power. Through his Internet site (www.franciscocontreras.com), his magazine *(Health Ambassador)* and interviews on television and radio, Dr. Contreras shares the prevention and treatment wisdom with all who desire to take charge over cancer. He travels constantly, speaking at conferences on cancer, because he believes that through proper education, cancer incidence and mortality can decrease.

In 1999 he traveled to Australia, New Zealand, China, Japan, Canada, the United States, Mexico, Paraguay, Jamaica, South Africa, Kenya, Austria and Russia. He truly goes to the extreme to share the knowledge and experience he has acquired through his medical practice.

Dr. Francisco Contreras is now personally reaching out to you to share how to gain victory over cancer. This landmark book gives you a comprehensive overview of what cancer is, the devastation it has caused, the successes and failures of cancer treatments and research and an in-depth look at both conventional and alternative treatment modalities. You will learn not only what factors lead to cancer, but also the practical things you can do to help prevent cancer from striking you or a loved one. Through redefining health, illness and victory over cancer, Dr. Contreras will lead you on a spiritual journey to assess who you are and what is truly valuable in life.

Introduction

The first few people who read this book called me to let me know how much it helped them overcome their fear of cancer. Dr. Francisco Contreras will help you put cancer in its place. If you have cancer, or if you are like everyone else and want to prevent it, this book will be one of the most important books you will ever read.

I have had the unique opportunity of working with Dr. Contreras and his father, Dr. Ernesto Contreras, Sr., for more than six years. I know them on a professional level and a personal level—Ernesto is my grandfather, and Francisco is my uncle. It has been my privilege to share in their mission to stop the suffering through education and compassionate therapies.

I witnessed Dr. Francisco Contreras graciously accept the appointment from his father to take the lead of this mission, and it is a honor to work alongside Francisco, a man of integrity, commitment and compassion. He has poured his heart, mind and soul into this book with the hope of helping every reader live the highest quality of life humanly possible. May you be blessed by this book as I have been.

—DANIEL E. KENNEDY
EXECUTIVE VICE PRESIDENT, OASIS OF HOPE HOSPITAL
FOUNDER AND CHAIRMAN, WORLDWIDE CANCER PRAYER DAY

Section I:
The Power of Hope

1

Is There Hope for Living Cancer Free?

SITTING IN A plush waiting room, Laura Red scanned the expressions of those who were lined up around her. Desperation and pain filled every face. She choked as she swallowed the panic that hardened into a knot in her throat. She wanted to announce loudly: *I don't belong here—I'm not one of you!*

Fidgeting in her chair, she rehearsed endlessly the details of the last few weeks as if the outcome might be different. First there had been the stomach pain, then the initial doctor visit. Then came the next evaluation and the series of medical procedures. Lots of names of syndromes and diseases had been thrown at her—viral infection, chronic fatigue syndrome, colitis, food poisoning. But the doctors couldn't settle on one.

In desperation, Laura herself suggested cancer, but a specialist assured her that she didn't have the "C" word. As time wore on, however, the resolve of the doctors faded, as more and more stern faces examined her. One of the faces along the way—she could no longer remember which one of countless specialists—had suggested a visit to this renowned oncologist, or cancer specialist. Convincing herself it was just one more step in the process of elimination, she submitted to more tests. Now she sat in his waiting room—a room with the walls closing in—waiting to hear the results.

As her eyes darted from one cancer patient to the next, horror filled her mind. She was sitting among the Nazi concentration camp prisoners she'd seen in films.

Just this morning the headlines read: "Cancer Epidemic in America." Was she going to become the newest member of this unfortunate group? It couldn't be possible! Laura was in the prime of life—twenty-nine years old, married (happily!) with four wonderful children: her firstborn daughter, twin sons, then another daughter to round the family out. This could not be happening! Surely she would wake up from this nightmare. Today in this very office, her story would have a happy ending.

Even if it is cancer, she conceded to herself, *it has to be in a very early stage. The symptoms aren't that bad.* She would be a disciplined patient, one to prove the statistics wrong.

"Laura Red, please come in."

The nurse's voice shook her out of her thoughts. After a curt introduction, the doctor snapped off a businesslike statement of her condition without looking up from his clipboard. "The cancer in your pancreas has already spread to your liver . . ."

Laura felt all the blood drain from her face, her neck, her arms. Lightheaded, she grabbed her chair for support. The doctor's words fell into slow motion. She struggled to focus on what he was saying.

" . . . three or four months to live. There is no time to waste. If you start the comprehensive chemotherapy program immediately, you could live six to twelve months. I've already made arrangements for you to have a CT-guided needle biopsy in two days to determine the type of cancer."

She could only distantly hear his words. Details of vomiting, pain, hair loss and other dreadful symptoms were hanging somewhere in the room.

Laura could not remember leaving the doctor's office or driving home. But by the time her husband, Joe, got home from work, she thought she had pieced herself together and hoped she could talk to him intelligibly. Instead she just collapsed into his arms and wept.

Two days later, Laura gathered her resolve. Whatever it took, she would do. She wanted to live.

A Relentless Epidemic

LAURA IS NOT alone. Every twenty-four seconds of every minute of every hour of every day, someone like Laura in America is confronted with the diagnosis of cancer. The American Cancer Society estimated that 1.2 new cancers were expected in 1999.[1] Every day, millions around the world face malignancies that threaten their lives and their families' well-being.

In one way or another, almost everyone is affected by cancer. As we move into a new millennium, 50 percent of men and 30 percent of women in the United States are expected, at some point in their lives, to have some form of cancer. Cancer is the second leading cause of death, exceeded only by heart disease. In the United States, one out of every four deaths is from cancer.[2]

The Advice of a Veteran

LAURA KNEW THE statistics, but they had seemed remote, unimportant—something for other people to worry about. Now the numbers were terrifyingly real. She pulled herself together and decided that she was not going to allow this enemy to control her. Surely in this advanced technological age science could conquer anything. She determined to declare war on this cancer with the power of the most advanced therapies on the globe and with the strength of her positive attitude.

When she returned to the oncologist for a second visit, Laura hid in a book, refusing to acknowledge her gaunt peers. The thought of becoming one of them was too appalling. They might all die—but she would live. Laura would beat it.

But one of the unacknowledged concentration camp victims was staring at her with a piercing look she could not avoid. Abruptly, he introduced himself as Robert and asked, "What's your diagnosis?"

Strange question, she thought. *Everyone else who knows about my cancer has said I am the picture of health.* "How did you know I had cancer?" she retorted.

"Are there any other reasons to see an oncologist?" His reply cut her to the heart.

"Well, I'm here to be cured of pancreatic cancer—there are no two ways about it." Laura studied her inquisitor. He was thin and ashen, not unlike the rest of the people there. His shirt hung loosely on him, the only trace of a rounder, more muscular frame. Laura softened a little and politely asked him about his well-being, even though it was obvious he was extremely ill. Robert replied with a load of unsolicited advice.

"Don't let them fool you," the veteran counseled. "The doctors said my cancer was not aggressive and that I had a very good chance of being cured because they 'caught it early.'

"I went by the book completely. I submitted to their scientifically proven program. I underwent radical, disabling surgery—and I came out with flying colors. Then, before I even could begin to recuperate, the oncologist recommended radiation to kill whatever malignant cells were 'left behind.'

"After the radiation, I was considered in 'remission'—that's the closest they come to saying 'cancer free.' Still I was offered chemotherapy as a preventative measure to increase my chances of cure. Little did I know that it would be so devastating. It may have destroyed any residual cancerous cells in my body, but it almost killed me in the process. I endured six months of torture. I vomited so much I had to be hospitalized. My hair fell out. I didn't want to eat or even live. The chemo felt worse than the cancer. But I endured it because it was going to make me better. And I recuperated well.

"I was scheduled to come for follow-up once a month for three months, then the visits would only be every three months. I had beaten cancer!"

Laura had been politely listening to Robert's rambling, trying to ignore the unpleasant details. But that last statement about beating cancer got her attention. "If you have beaten cancer, then what are you still doing..." she began, but Robert interrupted by just continuing his story.

"One year after my diagnosis—nine months after the preventative chemo—I was finally feeling myself again. My hair had grown back—and without the gray! The specialist said that if everything continued to go well, my next visit could be put off for one year.

"I celebrated with my family and thanked God and everybody and everything else I could. Summer had just begun, and I planned to enjoy my second chance at life.

"Then the dreaded call from the nurse came. Apparently something was wrong with one of my blood tests. A tumor marker was elevated. She reassured me that it was probably a mistake, but they needed me to come in to repeat the test to make sure.

"The new test showed the marker even higher than before. The doctor wanted a new CT scan. I reminded him that three months ago all the scans and tests were negative. But he said he wanted to do some more anyway.

"It turned out that the elevated antigens—that's the tumor marker..." Robert paused for a second and added sympathetically, "You'll learn all these terms soon enough." Then he went right back into his discourse. "The tumor marker was in my liver. Three spots were found—the smallest was the size of a pea, and the largest was the size of a big marble.

"I was not prepared for any of this. The doctors wasted no time in telling me that I had to start chemotherapy immediately, or else I would not be celebrating Christmas! But I had already gone through chemotherapy, and I wanted no more of it. So I talked to my doctor about what my chances would be if I did nothing."

Laura was all ears, waiting to hear how the doctor responded.

"My doctor said I'd be taking my life into my own hands—that I should think about my family and at least do what I could to fight it. So I reluctantly went along with more chemo.

"After the chemo, a new CT scan revealed that not only had the tumors grown considerably, but also new metastases had appeared in spite of the chemotherapy. Since the chemotherapy had failed, nothing else could be done. The doctor told me to get my affairs in order and enjoy whatever time I had left.

"Two rounds of chemotherapy and one of radiation— that's all it took to erase my quality of life. My tumor seems to grow by the day and along with it the pain. I'm depressed, and I'm sure you can tell that I'm frustrated and angry. Every time I look at my wife I feel such sadness, then I get scared, then the anger rises up. I need more and more morphine to bear the pain. I live between my cry for life and my body's wish for death."

Robert paused and looked reflective for a moment. "Cancer rules. You may knock it down, but you can't knock it out. It is foolish to be optimistic—that's a waste of time and your family's money. As I expected from the beginning, there is no hope."

Then Robert abruptly turned from her. Obviously the conversation was over. Laura was left there, standing in a river of painful emotion, hurt and anger that he had vented—and the knowledge that it could very soon be hers as well.

YES, WE HAVE NO BANANAS!

AS A DOCTOR and a CEO, I occasionally attend seminars to learn things that might improve our hospital's performance. At a recent total quality management seminar, I was listening to a man who was an expert in techniques used for putting clients at ease when the nature of your business has obvious short-comings. Well, the nature of my business definitely has shortcomings: Not everyone gets well!

This expert noted, "In a comfort-demanding society, where the client is always right, you must never give a negative outlook to your potential client lest you provoke his displeasure and rejection." Instead, he suggested approaching the problem head-on in a positive, proactive manner. I was with him that far. Then he presented his so-called "positive response" to a problem, which was saying, "Yes, we have no bananas!" I have to admit, the optimist in me was profoundly impacted by the simplicity—and stupidity—of this concept.

For many decades oncologists and patients alike have been hoping for that just-around-the-corner cancer cure promised since the beginning of this century, but even more earnestly since the official declaration of war against cancer in the seventies. Yet at the end of the most progressive century in history, society is still left wanting. Even the most fervent supporters of this scientific effort are questioning the value of the research. The response from the highest cancer authorities is still, "Yes, we have no bananas!" The tone is positive, and the first word we hear is "Yes!" But the end result is still "no bananas."

A MALEVOLENT FOE

CANCER BEGINS THROUGH genetic mutations that are caused either by errors in the normal wear and tear of cell reproduction or external aggressors such as chemicals. These mutated cells are similar to fast-growing embryonic cells. The difference is that cancer cells stay immature. Instead of growing just until they mature into an "adult" state, they continue to grow and grow. They are not typical in structure and do not have specialized functions.

This uncontrolled growth eventually invades surrounding tissue and, in most cases, sends clusters of cells from the mother tumor to other parts of the body via the lymphatic or circulatory systems (a spreading of the cancer called "metastasis"). So the cancer forms a parasitic relationship with the organism. In order to survive, it consumes the host and eventually kills it. When you have cancer, your body becomes the host of these destructive parasitic cancer cells.

So, why has cancer defeated the scientific techniques designed to defeat it? Man has effectively resolved incredible obstacles in the computer industry, electronics, physics, math and microbiology—we've even sent men to the moon and brought them back again. Why can't science solve the cancer puzzle?

I believe one reason is that cancer has the unique ability to adapt to the most inhospitable conditions and still survive, grow and disseminate. In addition, cancer has many causes. But we'll go into that more in the next section.

This formidable foe has mocked the best and most brilliant

minds in the world with its ability to elude predictable patterns. Cancer has no honor; it fights dirty, scorning the rules of scientific method.

Cancer patients like Laura, Robert and millions more face this unfair fight in their daily struggle against this monster, which respects neither age, sex, culture, religion nor social status.

Robert died quietly a few weeks before Laura decided to seek my help and treatment at Oasis of Hope Hospital. He had put everything about his life in order, down to the socks he wore in his coffin. (He didn't want them to clash with his favorite tie or with the coffin's lining.)

Laura read his obituary, remembering the last thing he said to her at a chance meeting in the hallway of the medical building. "It's my destiny," he had said. "All the prayers in the world would not change anything. Believe me—I've been there, done that. And what happened? My tumor is bigger every time they check it.

"The sane thing to do is to get your affairs in order—life insurance, the mortgage, loans and the funeral. At least since I stopped the chemotherapy, I feel good enough to do that."

Robert's words troubled her for days. Sadness for Robert and his family filled Laura's head. But more than that, his death underscored fear and doubt as to what course of action to take for herself.

AN ALTERNATIVE CHOICE

I REMEMBER THE day a vivacious and mischievous four-year-old ran into my office, touching everything. Fortunately, her mother, Laura Red, distracted her with crayons and a coloring book. Laura and her husband, Joe, related their story, hoping I could be of help.

It had been a few months since her first encounter with

cancer, and the blanket of sorrow surrounding her was almost tangible. Some remnant of her beauty was still appreciable in her demeanor. A turban covered her hairless head, and heavy makeup tried to mask her hollow cheeks. She moved deliberately, like an old woman, and her furrowed brow betrayed her constant pain.

"If I had listened to Robert," she said regretfully, "I would have not opted for all the aggressive treatment that devastated my quality of life and left me hopeless. I don't want to die, but I have to admit that this monster is bigger than science and technology. My fighting strength is belittled by its power."

Laura was an educated woman who had always subconsciously believed in the abilities of modern advancements to conquer problems. She studied everything she could about her enemy, and now she had information overload. Some of the information was easy to grasp; some of it was confusing and even contradictory. And none of it contained the answer she hoped to find.

The odds that more chemotherapy and radiation would succeed were low. The best they could offer was a few more months with a lot less quality of life. So Laura made a firm decision to commit to alternative therapy. She changed her diet, her attitude and even her beliefs.

As Laura's cancer progressed, her faith in science failed her. "Life-and-death situations call for all the help you can get," she reflected. "It feels funny—and empty—to call out to 'chance' to help you. In spite of all my reservations about God, it just makes more sense to call on Him for help. I'll pray however long it takes for a miracle. What do I have to lose?"

Although she didn't want to leave her children motherless as young as they were, Laura also confessed to me (with shame) that she was plain terrified to die, so she was putting up this fight for herself as well.

I understood her moral anguish. "Life is impossible to live

without some selfishness," I reassured her. "Remember, the airline attendants tell you that, in the event of a mishap, you should put on your own oxygen mask first and then attend to your children. This is not selfish; it's just plain common sense. You get healthy, and then you'll be better able to help your husband and children."

Still she wondered about the fight, the investment, the anguish, the times away from her children. The financial strain of this monster had all but depleted the children's college fund. Was all this work, sorrow and sacrifice really worth the effort? Or was Robert right after all?

HOPE FOR LIVING CANCER FREE

THE ODDS SEEM overwhelmingly against people with cancer. Every minute that ticks by, one patient dies from cancer in America alone—that is about 560,000 who will die this year in America, the most technologically advanced country in the world.[3] And millions succumb to cancer each year worldwide. Paradoxically, it seems that the more we know about cancer, the more people fall victim to it.

Is there really hope of living cancer free in this day and age? Is there hope of preventing cancer from ruining so many? Is there hope for those who have already fallen prey to its devastating hold?

Yes, I believe we can liberate ourselves from cancer—and that's not foolish, optimistic rhetoric. There truly is hope of living cancer free. I have found that we can fall victim to cancer, or we can rise victorious above it. And for the most part, it is a matter of choice!

Allow me through this book to introduce you to an arsenal of breakthrough strategies that can empower you to liberate yourself from cancer's grip. Preventing cancer before it hits is the most effective way of being cancer free. But when prevention is no longer an option, it's never too late to counter or even to conquer cancer.

Allow me to share with you my experiences with effective breakthrough strategies, both orthodox and unorthodox. These therapies don't merely fight tumors; they also address the body, soul and spirit, and they provide physical, emotional and spiritual resources that empower people to triumph in this life-and-death battle—just as Laura did.

LAURA'S NEW LIFE

LAURA BEGAN ALTERNATIVE therapy. Weeks passed, then months, then years. At the writing of this book, it has been nine years since Laura was first diagnosed with cancer. She has since enjoyed a full life with her children, and most likely she'll enjoy her grandchildren's weddings.

About a year ago she decided to visit the oncologists who had "prophesied" her doom. She wanted to share her good news. As you can imagine, they were surprised to see her. The medical staff reviewed her case and requested a battery of tests, none of which showed cancer. Laura was elated, and she graciously shared with them her experience with alternative therapies. She also thanked God for her miracle.

"Maybe you should look into this avenue of treatments," she suggested to the oncologist.

"Laura," he said, "I am sorry, but there is no treatment on earth that can cure advanced cancer of the pancreas."

"So, what happened to me?"

"Well," the doctor began, "it is not uncommon to make diagnostic mistakes. We believe that our pathologist misdiagnosed you. Most likely you had chronic pancreatitis that resolved itself. The 'tumors' you had must have been inflammatory tissue, and the enlarged lymph nodes resolved with the control of the infection you probably had. This is the most plausible explanation for what you are calling a 'miracle.'"

Laura was shocked. "Are you telling me that I never had cancer, that you gave me radiation and chemotherapy—treatments that threatened my life—that I didn't even need?"

"Medicine is not perfect. Errors are made," the doctor replied flatly.

Laura was understandably upset that the doctor dismissed her experience and her healing. She immediately called me, confused and angry.

I listened sympathetically. Of course, it was not the first time I had heard such a story. By this stage in life, I have developed a tragic sense of humor about the blindness of those in my own medical profession. So I comforted Laura with this story:

> An agnostic tried to dissuade a Bible believer by saying, "The 'miracle' of the Red Sea is a farce. At the time of Moses, the Red Sea was at most a couple of feet deep!"
>
> "Wow," the believer replied, "then there was more than one miracle, and it was even greater than I thought!"
>
> "What do you mean?" asked the puzzled agnostic.
>
> "Well, not only did God part the Red Sea, but all those Egyptians drowned in such shallow water!"

Laura laughed.

"Laura, let me tell you that it is not easy to make the kind of mistake in diagnosis they are talking about," I reassured her. "Chronic pancreatitis never—I repeat, *never*—gives liver metastasis, and that metastasis was very clear in your CT scan. "But," I added, "even granting that possibility, then God cured you of chronic pancreatitis, which is still a good miracle!"

Today Laura is thirty-eight and cancer free. Let's find out how it was possible.

2

Breakthrough
Strategies

How did Laura Red achieve such a miraculous recovery? She worked hard to prepare for it by using every resource at her disposal.

Success always depends upon resources. Some people succeed because of their financial resources, others because of the sharpness of their minds, others just by their brute physical strength. The more balanced people are in these three areas, the better their chances for success.

During an interview a few years ago, Barbara Walters asked John F. Kennedy, Jr., if he felt pressured to be successful because of his Kennedy heritage. He could have answered with a simple yes or no, but he didn't. Instead, he said something like, "We must take advantage of all the resources given to us." The profoundness of his response impacted me. He chose to acknowledge that he had the responsibility to be a good steward of the resources given to him. No more. No less.

First World countries have achieved a great level of comfort for themselves by using their resources. But those resources have also been exploited at times and have harmed the environment.

Although as a nation we Mexicans have not taken advantage of all our resources, we do have a sense of "enoughness" that makes sanity and happiness a priority over achievement and material surplus. I believe we all need such a balance for our physical, emotional and spiritual well-being, both communal and personal.

PATIENTS NEED INFORMATION

YEARS OF PRACTICE and thousands of interviews have helped sensitize me to patients' individual needs. Some may need pampering, others firmness to help them get in line with their programs. But all patients want me to explain to them their course of treatment. They all want to understand the actions and reactions of the medication; they also want to know what this is for and what that is for; they want a clarification of their prognosis. Regardless of personality, culture or academic background, they all want information, information and more information.

Doctors in general are "communicationally challenged." I'm sure this is not news to you. We doctors spend too little time with our patients, and we talk to them—or rather, at them—in a foreign language. This causes the patient to feel belittled and fearful. A patient like this goes into the therapy program unaware and ignorant, and thus becomes a unhelpful team member in the healing process. I believe that the more informed an individual is, the better he or she will cooperate with the treatment and respond to it.

Often individuals will reject therapies that they are not convinced are best for them. I have learned to respect a person's right to make decisions such as this as long as I'm sure they have enough facts to be responsible. I encourage patients to ask questions and to be active participants in the doctor's office and in the hospital room. A knowledgeable person is the best ally in the adventure of healing.

Breakthrough Strategies

TREATING PATIENTS, NOT CANCER

AS WE WILL explore in this book, the fight for a cancer cure is being fiercely waged in the most avant-garde medical research centers and universities of the richest countries of the world. If all that talent, money and technology have not yet solved the cancer puzzle, it is reasonable to assume we are doing something wrong.

We are searching in the wrong direction.

Conventional cancer treatment focuses on destroying the tumor. At first, this seems the obvious route to take. But almost one hundred years of trials prove otherwise. If surgically removing, irradiating or chemically dissolving tumors, although somewhat effective, has not lowered cancer death rates in any part of the world, should we not try something else?

In my practice I refuse to treat cancerous tumors; instead, I choose to treat individuals. This cliché is as old as medicine, but it is rarely applied. Since cancer—or any disease, for that matter—is the failure of the body to maintain proper functions due to poor management, loss or lack of resources, my mission is to provide my patients with the resources necessary for them to heal themselves. It's a simple statement, but it's worth repeating. With the right resources, our bodies can heal themselves.

RESOURCES FOR TOTAL HEALTH

EVERY CREATURE HAS the capability of regenerating itself at the cellular level, which is why creation has no spare parts hanging around. This applies to humans as well, and I believe it is by design, not chance. The liver replaces 100 percent of its cells about every three months. Some blood cells are reproduced every eight minutes. Our bodies are constantly reproducing cells to replace dying ones.

The Hope of Living Cancer Free

In order for people to regenerate themselves, resources must be provided to the whole person—body, mind and spirit. Patients who fare the best are those who have been able to store up resources.

Although I am a cancer specialist and have acquired knowledge in this field, I am humbled by the complexity of cancer. Yet in my efforts to truly help people, I have found there is a much more successful way to help my patients than typical intervention: I guide them to identify what resources their bodies, minds and spirits need both to recuperate and then to preserve total health. Here is a list of some of those resources:

PHYSICAL	MENTAL/EMOTIONAL	SPIRITUAL
Food	Family relationships	Relationship with God
Pharmaceuticals	Friends	Prayer
Vitamins/minerals	Counselors	Faith
Good living environment	Meditation	Biblical healing words
Exercise	Stress management	Confession
Knowledge	Knowledge	Knowledge
Wisdom	Wisdom	Wisdom

Let's take a brief look at a few of these resources, starting with the tangible ones. By the way, this isn't the last you'll be hearing about these. Not only are they critical for intervention, but also for prevention, which is the very best cure!

Most modern illnesses, with the exception of inherited ones, are the products of both our behavior and the quality of our environment. The most common causes of death are cardiovascular diseases, cancer, diabetes, obesity, infections and accidents. Determining factors in these include things we can control—cigarette smoking, alcoholism, bad eating habits and destructive working conditions. In other words, we can provide ourselves with better resources.

Breakthrough Strategies

A *healthy diet*

In the United States, a high percentage of fatalities (heart attacks, cancer, cerebrovascular accidents, diabetes and obesity) are directly related to lifestyle.[1] Hippocrates said, "Let your food be your medicine and your medicine your food." Unfortunately, we have acquired the terrible habit of eating the convenient, fast "un-foods" and junk "un-foods."

In 1994 it was reported that 25 percent of the Mexican population suffered from malnutrition while 70 percent of the population was obese.[2] Those figures seem contradictory, but they both reflect improper nutrition. Because of that, disorders that were considered eradicated in other countries, such as some skeletal and cardiovascular problems, were on the increase in Mexico.

Insurance companies charge premiums directly proportional to the body weights of their clients. In other words, they fine obesity simply because obese people have a greater risk of dying of heart attacks, cancer, cerebral embolism and diabetes.

We all need good food to maintain optimum health. When we eat right, we are healthier—in our bodies and our minds. One recent study done in the state of New York demonstrated that well. The administration of public schools in New York, together with the state government, removed all the foods offered at the school cafeteria that had artificial color and flavor additives, as well as other types of additives and preservatives. They also significantly reduced products with sugar and refined flour.

The study concluded that the one million students in New York's 803 public schools raised their grades an average of 39 to 54.9 percent during the length of the study.[3] Not a single change was made in the curriculum or in the human resources team. These impressive statistics were a direct result of the changes in the diet during school hours. The scientists who carried out the study concluded that if changes had been extended to the diet at home, the results would have been extraordinary.

Another series of studies made at youth detention centers involved 8,076 youngsters from twelve correctional centers. Chemical additives, sugar and refined flour were withdrawn from their diets. At the end of these studies, the aggressive and destructive behaviors of the detained youngsters diminished 47 percent.[4]

In Virginia, 276 young detained delinquents with a severe criminal background were given a healthy diet for two years. During that period jail theft declined 77 percent, insubordination 55 percent and hyperactivity 65 percent.[5]

Another healthy food study in Los Angeles involved 1,382 teenage offenders. Again, the results were positive. There was a reduction of 44 percent in their delinquent behaviors and suicide attempts.

The above studies demonstrate that when youngsters (and adults) follow a healthy diet—including highly nutritious foods such as vegetables, fruits and cereals, and excluding refined sugar, artificial colors, flavor additives and chemical preservatives—both physical and mental health improve.

I have observed that poor eating habits and lifestyles are passed on from generation to generation effortlessly, while change through education is a slow process at best. So I am making my best effort to let people know that disease starts in the mouth. If you don't watch what you are putting in it, you will get sick. Nutrition is the chief ally of health.

Vitamins and minerals

We need vitamins and minerals because we never take in enough of the right foods to obtain the substances needed to prevent disease. Vitamins are nutrients that are not proteins, carbohydrates, fats or minerals. They improve metabolism, prevent disease and help slow the aging process.

The human body doesn't have the power to extract minerals directly from the environment or to manufacture them from other substances. Our only source of minerals is food. Of the elements most important for our organs to function and survive, minerals are at the top of the list.

Exercise

A little exercise goes a long way. It doesn't take a lot to make a difference. To keep yourself in good physical condition you should, on average, walk briskly from twenty-five to sixty minutes three times a week. That's not asking much!

Exercise reduces chemical stress in our bodies by the neutralization of acids. It also improves mental agility and memory, and it rehabilitates disturbances of the nervous system. It improves posture, reduces dysfunction of the joints and strengthens the bones.

The digestive system is aided by exercise in that it helps prevent constipation. Exercise also improves the efficiency of the heart and lungs, increases circulation, reduces cholesterol and strengthens the immune system. It also helps in reducing depression and lifting the spirits.

Living environment

A good living environment has a positive impact, not only on physical health, but also on emotional and spiritual health. Let me give you an example here. Sometimes a child who is hyperactive may be thought to have an emotional problem when, in fact, he truly has an allergy to something in the house. The child is unaware of the allergy or the cause of his discomfort, but through his behavior he subconsciously sends out a signal to his parents that something is wrong. It can be difficult, but if the parents can discover the physical thing to which their child is allergic and remove it, the child may no longer be hyperactive.

We see this all the time. A depressed person may not have as many emotional or spiritual problems as one might think at first. The depression may be a simple vitamin deficiency. Give that person the vitamin he needs, and his depression goes away.

If you can create a good living environment where you feel at peace, you will see physical, emotional and spiritual problems diminish.

Well, perhaps all this makes sense to you. After all, we know that we need good food and clean air to live. We may even admit needing exercise. But what about the less tangible items, such as knowledge, relationships and faith? Do we really need these resources to maintain health?

I have discovered that yes, we do. Let's find out how they help.

Stress management

We can experience physical, emotional and spiritual stress independently or in combinations. For this reason, we need to employ stress-management techniques for each area. Physical stress is anything that is taxing our bodies, such as heat, weight or resistance. The best way to manage this type of stress is to move away from the stressor or employ something to counteract it. For example, if heat is getting to you, you can move out of the sun or put up an umbrella to create shade.

Emotional stress may be more difficult to identify. It may be caused by deadlines at work, economic problems, domestic tension or, worst of all, unfocused anxiety. It is important to communicate to others and develop trust relationships in which you can "let someone in" to walk your path with you. Exercise is also an effective way to relieve emotional stress.

Spiritual stress generally results when physical or emotional stress becomes unmanageable, and it eats right through to our souls. Doubt and fear dominate us, and the questions of who we are and why we exist go unanswered. I find that prayer, fasting and fellowship with spiritually strong people help me during these times.

Unresolved stress, be it physical, emotional or spiritual, can manifest itself in physical illness. That's why it's important to manage stress now.

Positive attitude

It is not the clothes that make the person; it is what he thinks in his heart. Many patients I have watched beat cancer have had a positive attitude. The things we declare with our mouths often come true. The self-fulfilling prophecy is real. If you declare that cancer will end your life, it probably will. Be positive with your words daily, telling yourself and others that you are getting well. The rest of your body will strive to comply with your positive words.

Relationships

Relationships are so important. So many of my patients who have breast cancer have expressed that they feel unloved by their husbands. I tell husbands that they can help prevent breast cancer by loving their wives and encouraging them.

Humans need love to live. Life can easily slip away. Enjoy each relationship you have, whether with a sibling, coworker, spouse or child. If you gain the whole world but have not love, what does it profit you?

The doctor-patient relationship is critical for healing to take place. If you are a patient, you need to communicate everything you are feeling or experiencing to your doctor. At first, he may not know what to do with so much information from you, but it will help him as he is trying to uncover what you really need.

Knowledge and wisdom

Laura Red is well today because she decided to take advantage of the resources she had, to pursue the ones she lacked and to utilize all of them wisely to restore her natural defense mechanisms, which were designed to destroy any threatening aggressor, including cancer.

Too good to be true? It's good, and it's definitely true. It's also simple, though it is not necessarily achieved without effort. Getting rid of cancer often depends on how informed a patient is.

Wouldn't it be nice for life's complicating moments to arrive at convenient times? Why is it that diseases in general arrive at the worst possible time? Because they do, it is important to become informed now about the best therapeutic approaches—orthodox and alternative. That includes general therapies as well as those for a specific type of cancer.

But most of us hate to spend money or time to inform ourselves about health issues—especially those we fear anyway. If you think knowledge is expensive, try ignorance. The Bible says that we are destroyed for lack of knowledge. (See Hosea 4:6.) I believe that's true.

Many cancer patients and their families are usually unaware of the alternatives until they realize that the established oncological therapies have failed, that "nothing more can be done." Only when patients find themselves against the wall do they start looking for options, and this search can become frantic and unwise. People who are desperate will grasp at straws, and there are plenty of charlatans out there. It's worth it to become informed *now*.

When cancer strikes, most oncologists recommend the most advanced treatment options based on the latest scientific research. But most of us experts fail to tell our patients that the latest, most advanced treatments provided in state-of-the-art oncological centers are quite ineffective.

Breakthrough Strategies

Often patients are unaware that alternative options exist, and their doctors rarely tell them. For instance, most patients won't be made aware that it has been scientifically and statistically proven that patients with some forms of cancer live longer and better if they reject any kind of aggressive therapy, such as radiation or chemotherapy.[6]

No one is more interested in you than you. Choosing the correct timing and order of existing therapies can be a matter of life and death. Empower yourself with knowledge that will help you and your doctor do what is best for you. Do not allow circumstances or the flow of events to carry you. When expectations fall short, desperate "what ifs" torment you. So take charge.

When we are prepared, we have better luck. Let me explain.

Many inventions and developments were hit upon by chance, but isn't it interesting that these "chance" developments usually happened to the researchers in the field—not the John Does on the street? You must know what you are doing in order to appreciate the opportunity that "chance" drops on your lap. "Chance," said Louis Pasteur, the famous French microbiologist, "favors the prepared minds."

In other words, educated preparation is a magnet that attracts "chance" breakthrough developments. If you want chance to come your way, be prepared. If you want a miracle from God, be prepared.

Staying healthy begins with education. I believe that doctors should be the procurers more than the restorers of health. The more we educate, the less we have to intervene.

Laura Red made the best of the resources available to her—therapeutic, mental, emotional and spiritual. She was willing to take time to acquire knowledge and apply it with wisdom in her decision-making process. She was faced with overwhelming and often confusing data, but she pursued pertinent information diligently and then committed to following her program to success.

That's the mission of this book—to provide powerful in-depth information based on the latest research, ancient wisdom and the awesome testimonials from patients who have "been there, done that." We want to help and uplift you or your loved ones with spiritual fortitude that is unshakable, even when it appears that God makes no sense.

This brings us to a critical resource in the art of maintaining balance and good health—our own connection with God.

Relationship with God

Being "cured of cancer" is not the only way of being freed from its claws, its devastation and its control. I have learned from my patients that cancer affects people far beyond their physical bodies. The emotional stress is devastating to their souls, and it depresses their immune systems. Hopelessness, discouragement and desperation demolish personal relationships and even families.

But the resentment cancer can cause spiritually is the most destructive of all.

Unfortunately, patients seldom realize that when God seems farthest away, His love, mercy and salvation are as near to them as the whisper of a prayer. I have discovered that reconciling with God, or reinforcing existing spiritual bonds, is the strongest tool available to stimulate the immune system and healing.

Success against any adversity requires recognizing and facing the obstacles first. Then we can positively and optimistically utilize the resources at hand. It is an illusion to hope for a life without problems, but to ask God for help is both reasonable and wise.

At Oasis of Hope Hospital, patients get bodily resources,

yes. But they are also presented with the opportunity to receive Christ as their Savior, because He represents an inexhaustible fountain of resources. This is why patients with strong spiritual ties to God can better face disease.

Their relationship with God helps them deal with the initial rage, frustration and despair that all people experience when they discover they are suffering from a disease. They trust in God and have hope. They keep a positive spiritual attitude because they fortify themselves with prayer and by reading His Word. The patient who knows he is saved through the merits of Christ does not fear death, because he knows where he is going.

Many cast aside these concepts as simplistic, but they forget that all human beings in every culture and religion know intuitively that they are spiritually eternal. As a doctor, I am concerned about providing my patients with a good quality of life during their fleeting physical existence. But shouldn't I also be concerned about their eternal existence?

We often defeat disease, but sometimes it defeats us. However, the most powerful aspect of a strong relationship with God is the purpose and meaning individuals find for their lives, whether cured of cancer or not. One day, sooner or later, we will cross from this transitory life to another that has no end. We don't want any of our patients to depart without knowing that living in Christ is the best life, now and forever.

Laura Red is well today because she resolved to depend on the will of God for her future. Even before the tumors disappeared she claimed victory over cancer. She prayed, "Lord, if You heal me, I'll dedicate my life to bringing more people to You. However, if You don't heal me, I'm ready now to meet You in that place where there is no more sorrow or pain."

RESOURCES PROVIDE VICTORY

GRETA, AN ARDENT little Swedish patient, came to Oasis of

Hope Hospital for a consultation. She had a smile on her face that never vanished, and that precious smile has remained engraved in my mind since the first time I first saw her.

At the time Greta was fifty years old. In spite of her contagious energy and vitality, she had been sent home to die because she had "failed to respond" to surgery and chemotherapy for a cancer of the thyroid, which had metastasized to the lungs. This tumor was growing at a very fast rate. When several oncologists told her nothing else could be done, she decided to try "quackery," as she called it!

Greta related her story to me in her strong accent. The words came out of her mouth like bullets from a machine gun. "Doktor, I'm not greddy to retire!" she announced.

Greta was used to self-discipline, so she followed our prescribed program with precision. Every time she came for follow-up, the tumor in her lung was larger. But she would not falter. "Doktor, I'm not greddy to retire!" she would always say.

The tumor kept growing, then more tumors showed up in the lung, then tumors were in both lungs. Greta always came with the same attitude and the same smile. "Doktor, I'm not greddy to retire!"

After almost thirteen years of a miraculously excellent quality of life, she came to her appointment with a new decision and that typical smile. "Doktor, now I'm greddy to retire!" Greta lived successfully and comfortably with cancer for many years. Cancer didn't defeat Greta even though it finally took her life!

It may stun you to discover that individuals who have been sent home to die can live for years—even decades—with cancer. They just have to take full advantage of all the resources available to them—physical, therapeutic, mental, emotional and spiritual.

It is my goal to prepare you, through the wisdom of prevention, to fend off cancer before it begins; to qualify you to choose proper treatment options to combat cancer if you have it; and to pave the way for you to exercise full control in your quest for freedom from cancer.

But first, let's find out about disease in general—its causes and the treatments to combat it. I believe it will become clear that we all need a paradigm shift in our thinking about disease in order to win the battle against cancer.

3

Empowered Thinking

T HEY'VE POISONED THE wells. Let's kill them all!" That was the cry of thousands of Europeans in the mid-fourteenth century. The Black Death was spreading across the continent, killing millions, and many blamed it on a conspiracy by the Jews.

The word of this alleged treachery arrived in Strasbourg, Germany, which had so far been spared from the Black Death. The city officials tried to save the Jews, but they were deposed and a new government installed. On Valentine's Day, 1349, two thousand Jews were burned to death in a Jewish cemetery in Strasbourg.

However, those who blamed the Jews for this great plague discovered their error when the plague broke out in Strasbourg that summer, killing sixteen thousand.

People have always tried to find the causes of plagues, diseases and sickness. Some efforts have been tragically misguided; yet others have led to the discovery of cures.

Scientists have sacrificed their own lives and those of their families in their commitment to find cures for diseases that oppress society. Today, talented researchers and clinicians, supported by government coffers and private donations worldwide, are waging a vigilant battle against cancer.

New research avenues, amazing diagnostic tools, unique and exciting surgical techniques—all are the talk of the day in medical congresses the world over. From the most renowned research centers we are told that genetic engineering will bring the cure for cancer—even the replacement of limbs. Hope is always in the air. But hope has been in the air for a long time—with no results.

Industry today is totally dependent on technological advancements, which have improved every aspect of production, efficiency and development. Personal productivity today has probably increased a thousandfold since the beginning of the century. Just think about the amount of time a $20 calculator saves an engineer.

So the question is, How have the advances in the field of medicine benefited victims of cancer?

MONEY AND TECHNOLOGY— HOW HAVE THEY HELPED?

AMERICANS ARE OBSESSED with their health. No country in the world spends more money in the development of medical gadgetry than does the United States. Yet Americans are less healthy and less well-looked-after than other Westerners.[1]

At the beginning of the last decade of the millennium, the National Institute of Health estimated that the cost of cancer is $107 billion annually in the United States.[2] The cost of pain, emotional anguish and human life is, of course, incalculable.

"The United States operates a health care system that is unique among nations," declares an article published in the January 7, 1999, issue of the *New England Journal of Medicine.* "It is the most expensive of systems, outstripping over half again the health care expenditures of any other country."

According to the article, the primary reason for the increase in the health sector's share of the gross domestic product over the past thirty years is technological change in medicine. "America's trillion dollar health care system is vast—indeed, larger than the budgets of most nations—and it serves as a perpetual job-creating enterprise, providing employment to some nine million people," comments Arnold Relman, M.D., from Harvard. "Our medical care system grows ever more expensive, dysfunctional and inequitable."[3]

Are the goals of American medicine unrealistic? In his book *False Hopes: Why America's Quest for Perfect Health Is a Recipe for Failure,* Daniel Callahan, a philosopher and world-renowned bio-ethicist, says that "we have overemphasized the use of expensive technological innovation in return for only marginal gains."[4] The major hindrance to healthcare is an unrealistic faith in technology and overconfidence in the ability of medical science to eliminate illness and delay death, according to Callahan. "We need to realize that perfect health is unattainable, and we must be willing to limit our spending on medical care to keep it compatible with the needs for other essential social goods and services."[5]

In general, we all have the notion that medicine has come a long way. That's very true—the number of successes are as astounding as they are diverse. But we cannot overlook the cold fact that, for the most part, the failures obscure the successes. Of the approximately fifteen hundred diseases described in medical books, we only have cures for about twenty-three of them! For the rest, we can only hope for control of symptoms and delay of death at best, and even these come at the expense of quality of life.

More people are dying of cancer now than ever, even though we have more knowledge about cancer and more powerful and sophisticated therapeutic tools than ever. Despite decades of research and innumerable trials of new therapies, cancer remains a major cause of morbidity and mortality.

Believe me, I criticize my profession—the most ministerial of professions—with passionate love. I beg you not to forget the sacrifice, commitment and passion with which most physicians treat their patients. Even though there must be some out there, I do not know even one doctor who would willingly harm a patient. Why, then, are doctors failing at their goal of healing?

I strongly believe it has to do with the direction that the science of medicine has chosen to follow. Only a historical perspective can illuminate this erroneous path. Let's review, in a fast-forward mode, the fascinating birth of modern medicine and the events that preceded the introduction of the scientific method in the last one hundred years or so. It's a story of epic—or shall I say, epidemic—proportions.

HOW DID OUR THINKING ABOUT MEDICINE DEVELOP?

THROUGHOUT HISTORY, EPIDEMICS have killed a vast number of people. In the late Middle Ages the common epidemics were malaria, leprosy, typhus, influenza and St. Anthony's Fire. Perhaps the pestilence that desolated Europe the most was the Black Death, a bubonic plague of the pulmonary type. It began around 1333 in the central region of Asia and extended itself to the Mediterranean Sea, Russia and Ireland; it reached its climax in 1348. It is said that one-fourth of the population where it struck—twenty-five million people—died.

At the end of the fifteenth century, syphilis took on epidemic proportions, not respecting social class, rank or sex. Cholera claimed the lives of one hundred thousand

Frenchman in 1832. Typhus claimed three million Poles and Russians in 1914, followed by the flu epidemic that killed twenty-five million people in 1918.

The authorities used desperate methods to control epidemics. They burned corpses together with all their belongings. They even set entire cities ablaze, petitioned the heavens and offered all sorts of sacrifices. Jews were sometimes blamed and massacred by the thousands.

We can't begin to imagine what these people suffered during these epidemics. News from South America and Africa about the horrors of cholera or ebola offers but a vague hint.

In the seventeenth century, more new diseases were identified: rickets, tuberculosis and beriberi. Smallpox attacked Europe in the eighteenth century, but an important medical event contributed to the fight against it.

A NEW MEDICAL PARADIGM

EDWARD JENNER (1749–1823), a rural British doctor, came across a folk belief that people who contracted cowpox could not contract smallpox. Jenner made that idea the subject of experimentation for two years. Then in 1796, he injected secretions of cowpox into the arm of a child. Six weeks later he inoculated the youngster with the pus of smallpox. Absolutely no symptoms of smallpox showed up in the child—and immunization was born.

Immunization is based on the principle that individuals who survive a forced attack by a germ are protected from future attacks. Therefore, if a person is exposed to a light attack, he or she could be protected during an epidemic. Since Jenner's serum was obtained from cattle (or *vacca* in Latin), this method of immunization became known as a "vaccination."

Up to this time, scientists could do nothing but stand by

and watch as plagues took their toll. But the invention of the microscope and the discovery of the germ brought to light the causes of these devastating, infectious plagues. When doctors were able to look their enemies in the face, they realized that death did not come as a result of chance, divine judgment or the Jews.

With the enemy in sight, the fear of God was transferred to the fear of germs. Doctors, immunologists, microbiologists, physiologists and many other specialists waged war against an infinitely small but tremendously resourceful foe. Their scientific drive, restricted for so many centuries, emerged with a passionate force that could not be stopped. Physicians at last had the excited hope of achieving the victory over infectious diseases caused by these insolent, minuscule microbes.

TWO WAYS OF THINKING

TWO VERY DIFFERENT ways of thinking, or paradigms, emerged following the dramatic discovery of germs and the great hope it gave to medieval people. These two opposing schools of thought were headed by two gigantic figures—Claude Bernard and Louis Pasteur. In the matter of the method of disease development, what was black for one was white for the other.

The body's ability to heal itself depends upon its general condition—that is to say, how well-nourished it is, according to Claude Bernard (1813–1878), French physician and physiologist. Bernard believed that if the body had an adequate internal environment, it would know how to maintain the proper state of balance and health—no matter what germ it was exposed to.

Bernard concluded that germs are only responsible for the development of disease when the body offers conditions favorable to the germ, that is, a depleted state of health.

However, if the body maintains an adequate *milieu intérieur,* or internal environment, it will be able to fight off the germ and avoid disease.

It seemed like an irrefutable argument. How else could one explain the fact that, though we all come in contact with the same germs, only a few of us fall ill?

Bernard's theory was fundamental to the "humorist" school of thought. Of course, Bernard had a sense of humor, but the name "humorist" did not refer to that. It was assigned to give honor to Hippocrates who, five hundred years before Christ and without the help of microscopes, knew that there were "forces within us that truly heal." The ancient Greeks believed that the body was formed by four *humors* (Latin for "liquids"). Any alteration in their perfect balance caused pain, disease and even emotional changes; hence the modern reference to being in good or bad humor.

Louis Pasteur (1822–1895), however, disagreed with Bernard, asserting that germs were the true villains in disease, and that by neutralizing them, infections could be prevented and even cured. He proved his belief by his vaccines and treatments. This is the fundamental theory of the "causalist" school of thought, so named for its belief that if the cause of a disease can be determined, the saving antidote can be developed.

Pasteur's prestige was founded on his accomplishments in microbiology. The experiments he conducted confirmed that illness was the result of germs. Pasteur also demonstrated that germs reproduce themselves like any other organism. If these ideas sound familiar, it's because these advances formed the guiding principles of disease-control research. Today, many owe their lives to the achievements of Pasteur, even though the methods employed in his research were reckless. Pasteur frequently carried out experiments that were neither ethical nor humane.

One of his achievements was the vaccine against rabies. But with no more clinical data than Jenner had, Pasteur prepared the vaccine, gave it to a healthy volunteer and then infected him with rabies! Pasteur and his colleagues must have spent many anxious hours and days waiting for the deadly outcome, but the "guinea pig" survived and was declared successfully inoculated.

This experiment got everybody's attention and gave Pasteur even more notoriety than before in the eyes of scientists and the public. Soberly and humbly, and demonstrating the genius he was, Pasteur declared, "Chance favors the prepared mind."

One of the great misfortunes of being human is the fact that we spend so much time in the dark, waiting for the answers. So, when Pasteur finally turned on the light in the search for the illusive germ, almost everyone followed him and the causalist school of thought.

The French government funded a research institute so Pasteur could continue with the exploration of microorganisms. The Pasteur Institute, begun in 1886, to this date is at the forefront of scientific discovery. Their last great discovery was the human immunodeficiency virus (HIV).

When I think of Pasteur, I feel like a single brick lying beside the Sears Tower in Chicago, and I'm sure many of my colleagues feel the same. Pasteur and others were models of dedication. They truly laid down their lives for the pure joy of discovery.

Take, for example, Elie Metchnikoff (1845–1916), the Russian biologist and pathologist who discovered the white blood cells that attack any new invader. He later moved to Paris to be able to work with Pasteur and his institute. With the passing of the years he was able to absorb the "advances" in the struggle against infection, but his observations and research caused him to question Pasteur's theory that germs caused diseases. Eventually, he switched to Claude Bernard's humorist school of thought.

Metchnikoff and several coworkers stood before a group of physicians and drank a liquid contaminated with the deadly disease cholera. He wanted to prove the humorist's perspective that if the immune system is strong, it has the power to resist the germs. Few had paid attention to his work because Pasteur disagreed with it.

Metchnikoff's demonstration overwhelmed his colleagues when not a single one of the participants in the experiment fell sick with cholera. Although the course of history was not changed, Metchnikoff gained respect, so much so that Pasteur named him as his successor in 1904. Metchnikoff continued his studies in immunology and physiology, and he won the Nobel Prize for Medicine in 1908.

The search for new germs marched on. Robert Koch (1843–1910) discovered the two most feared germs of all time—those of tuberculosis and cholera. For that he received the Nobel Prize for his work in 1905. During that time germs were discovered that cause typhoid fever, gonorrhea, malaria, diphtheria, amoebiasis, tetanus, meningitis, syphilis and rubella.

THE SEARCH FOR
THE SILVER BULLET

SCIENTISTS SEARCHED FOR treatments that could destroy specific germs without damaging normal cells. This search for the "silver bullet" continues to be the guiding principle of the modern-day pharmaceutical industry.

The accidental discovery of penicillin, one of these silver bullets, occurred in 1928. Alexander Fleming (1881–1955), a British bacteriologist, had searched for the germs that caused the influenza epidemic of 1918, which killed twenty-five million people. Leaving for a holiday, he accidentally left his bacteria cultures on the work table in his London laboratory. When he returned he discovered that they had become contaminated with green fungus, which amazingly had destroyed the microorganisms of the culture. There is no doubt that "chance favors the prepared." This "chance" earned him the Nobel Prize in 1945.

Massive production of antibiotics began in the 1950s, and since then, doctors and researchers have not looked back. They have tirelessly devoted themselves to conquering the infectious and insolent bugs that cause diseases.

The success of antibiotics guaranteed that the causalist's school of thought would flourish. It has now become an immovable institution. Those who oppose it today are disregarded without so much as a backward glance, because this paradigm (or framework) of thinking is considered medical dogma.

But I have discovered from my work with thousands of patients that Bernard was correct—the internal environment in proper balance is what truly determines health.

BETTER LIVING CONDITIONS— THE OVERLOOKED HERO

DEVELOPING DRUGS THAT destroy germs and bacteria has benefited the world with better health, according to the medical industry. However, plagues and diseases have also been controlled through better hygiene, better distribution of food and city planning. Public health problems probably diminished in great measure because of these factors long before vaccinations were given.

It is difficult for us to imagine the deplorable living conditions of past centuries. Some time ago I read a book called *The Perfume* by Patrick Susskind. Though a novel, it describes with exquisite precision the environment of Paris in the eighteenth century. (If you are eating, I recommend you read this later.)

> In the period that interests us reigned stench scarcely conceivable to modern man. The streets reeked of manure, house yards stank of urine, halls and stairways smelled of rotting wood and rat excrement, kitchens were redolent of rotting cabbage and mutton fat, unventilated bedrooms stank of moldy dust, sleeping places smelled of greasy sheets, of humid quilts and the penetrating sweetish odor of urinals.
>
> The whole of the nobility stank and even the king stank like a carnivorous beast and the queen like an old goat; winter was no different than summer because in the 18th century they hadn't yet put a stop to the corrosive activity of bacteria and thus there was no human action, creative or destructive, no manifestation of life incipient or in decadence, that was not accompanied by some offensive odor.[6]

If the inhabitants of the most progressive city of Europe lived under such nauseating conditions, the plight of the rest of the Old World must have been unthinkable. In those miserable conditions, diseases spread like wildfire. Our immune systems, albeit incredibly resourceful, have limitations. When exposed to such unlimited bacterial onslaught, they can be unfairly challenged and fail.

Imagine that a doctor was thrown out of a hospital for suggesting that medical personnel wash their hands before treating patients. In 1847 Dr. Ignas Semmelweis was ousted from the University Hospital in Vienna for this "quackery." At that time doctors would do an autopsy and then, without washing their hands, deliver a baby! Of course, women with incredible immune systems survived, but those with any type of deficiencies succumbed to infections. Since pregnancy is accompanied by a physiological immune suppression in order for the mother not to reject the baby (a "foreign body"), many victims of the doctors' poor hygiene died.

By the way, my first daughter was born in this same hospital. Thank God that by that time they did wash their hands!

I believe we should let history speak for itself. Thanks to improvements in sewage and general sanitation, smallpox epidemics began to decline *before* Edward Jenner discovered the inoculation. Smallpox might actually have disappeared without any treatment at all. But doctors, pressured to respond to human suffering, popularized the general use of vaccination.

Curiously, the incidence of smallpox began to grow again toward the end of the nineteenth century: "After the use of cowpox vaccine became widespread in England, a smallpox epidemic broke out which killed 22,081 people. The smallpox epidemics became worse each year that the vaccine was used. In 1872, 44,480 people were killed by it. England finally banned the vaccine in 1948...Japan initiated compulsory vaccine in 1872. In 1892, there were 165,774 cases of smallpox there, which resulted in 29,979 deaths...Germany also instituted compulsory vaccination. In 1939 (this was during the Nazi regime), the diphtheria rate increased astronomically to 150,000 cases. Norway, which never instituted compulsory vaccination, had only fifty cases during the same period. Polio has increased 700 percent in states which have compulsory vaccination."[7]

CONQUEST OF TUBERCULOSIS CHART[8]

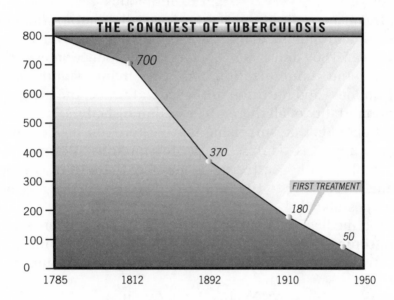

Another greatly feared epidemic in the nineteenth century was tuberculosis. As indicated by the preceding chart, in 1812 the death rate from tuberculosis in New York was 700 persons for every 100,000 inhabitants. By 1892 the rate had diminished to 370, and by 1910, to 180 per 100,000.[9]

Then in 1913 obligatory treatment began. Though in 1950 the rate stood at fifty per one hundred thousand, the need for the treatment has to be seriously questioned since the downward trend would probably have continued without the treatment.

Unfortunately, tuberculosis is on the rise again. You might think that people are better nourished and the conditions of our cities are better now than they were in the nineteenth century. Not necessarily so. The victims of tuberculosis are mainly the undernourished homeless who live in the slums of large cities in conditions that are as bad as those of the past century. To make matters worse, the modern tuberculosis germs are very resistant to antibiotics.

Infant mortality from scarlet fever, diphtheria, whooping cough and mumps diminished significantly all over Europe between 1869 and 1896[10]—before the introduction of antibiotics and immunization. As the living standards of cleanliness and nutrition improved in Europe, the incidence and mortality of all these diseases diminished.

It shouldn't be surprising that Pasteur, on his deathbed, was quoted as confessing to Metchnikoff, "Bernard was right. The pathogen [germ] is nothing; the terrain is everything," referring to the internal environment that Bernard had postulated.[11]

Yet, medical science did not change its course. The search continues for silver bullets that will do everything from destroying germs to curing cancer to keeping us young.

WE NEED A PARADIGM SHIFT

MORE THAN ONE hundred years of chasing silver bullets have not convinced scientists that the causalist school of thought offers only a mirage. But the paradigm has begun to shift.

Many medical authorities are now promoting radical but simple changes. Philip Lee, M.D., professor of social medicine and director of the health policy program at the University of California, San Francisco, went before the United States Senate in 1977 and warned the American people: "As a nation we have come to believe that technology can solve our major health problems...through the miracles of modern medicine. Appropriate public education must emphasize the unfortunate but clear limitations of current medical practice in curing the common killer diseases."[12]

Doctors are morally obligated to inform the public that the mission of medicine is much more than just intervention. We must educate society in the arena of prevention through lifestyle changes.

Medicine is an art. Sophisticated modern medicine has tried to convert the art of medicine into an exact science through technology and mechanization. In the eyes of my father, Dr. Ernesto Contreras, Sr., founder of Oasis of Hope Hospital, not to practice medicine as an art is a mortal offense to the Hippocratic Oath. He explained something to me about medicine that I will always keep with me.

> Until the nineteenth century, all the medical doctors in the world considered their profession a well-balanced mixture of art and science: the art of establishing a proper and beautiful doctor-patient relationship and the science of wisely using medical knowledge with a commitment to make progress.
>
> But unfortunately, in the twentieth century the science of medicine began to dominate over the art of medicine. Specialties and super-specialties were birthed. Now medical doctors have to dedicate so much time and effort keeping up to date on medical technology that they are not able to spend enough time on their relationships with their patients. The art is being left behind.
>
> This is more tragic in the practice of oncology, because at the present time, with a few exceptions, cancer specialists consider their practice to be purely scientific. This negligence is not only a philosophical or emotional problem. It has severely affected the rather poor results gained by the extremely aggressive and chilling practice of oncology during this century.
>
> It is imperative to return to the total care practice of oncology in which the oncologist treats not only the physical problem of the patient (the science of medicine), but

also the emotional, psychological and spiritual problems of each patient through a proper doctor-patient relationship (the art of medicine).

"Fantasy abandoned by reason produces monsters, but when united to it, is the mother of all art," said Francisco Goya, the famous Spanish artist. Medicine has to return to what it really is—first an art, and then, as a distant second, a science.

We must use wisdom to separate the hype from the hope. Reliance in knowledge and technology has been hyped since the beginning of the medical industry. But if we unite these with popular wisdom and common sense, the perspective for cancer control in the near future looks bright.

Now let's discover how medical science and its causalist approach to disease is faring in the modern war against cancer.

4

Hope for a Cure

L UNG CANCER THERAPY nearly perfected."
"Closing in on a cure for breast cancer."
"New hope for those with prostate cancer."
Springtime is a season of fresh hope. It is also the time
when excitement buzzes over possible new cancer cures in
the headlines and on the TV news—and it has been that way
for at least the last decade. This media explosion of new
hope always seems to coincide with the annual fund-raising
efforts of cancer education and research institutions.

For too long science has held out a carrot on a stick to
those devastated by cancer. I see the sad story repeated time
and time again in the lives of many cancer patients. Families
believe that the cure for cancer will be discovered just in time
to save their loved ones. Even when patients pass away, I
sometimes hear family members say, "If only he could have
hung on a little longer, then the cure might have been found."

There is hope for a cure, or rather for living cancer free.
However, based on science's track record, I don't believe it
lies with science and research. Decide for yourself as we

examine the modern battle against cancer.

The War on Cancer

ERADICATING CANCER IS the greatest challenge medical science has ever faced. No other disease has had more money or more hours of scientific study devoted to it. Since the 1920s when the United States government first funded studies on cancer, vast resources have been invested in the search for a cure. Regular reports of valuable discoveries have been the norm ever since.

I've been told that during World War II a ship called *Liberty,* which was carrying mustard gas, sunk. All the sailors had to jump into the water, where they were in contact with this mustard gas. Many died because of leukopenia, or the lowering of the white blood cell count. Since their white blood cells were depleted, their immune systems couldn't fight off sickness. They died of other complications, including many types of infections, especially pneumonia.

Someone at that time realized that maybe that gas or a derivative of it could be used for the cases of leukemia, in which the white blood cell count is extremely high. Therefore, the first drug that was developed was called mustargen. It was a big help for the children with some types of acute leukemia, as there was nothing that we could offer before that. The problem with that drug was its toxicity. Patients started vomiting and feeling terrible. But it was the only thing we had at that time, and it was excellent for leukemia and lymphomas.

After that, of course, the investigation into chemotherapy as a treatment for cancer started, and they were able to come up with the next drug, which was called cytoxin. That was the birth of the treatment of cancer with chemotherapy.

In 1955 a division of the National Institute of Health, the National Cancer Institute (NCI), established the Chemotherapy National Service Center (CNSC). This center appropriated $25 million to "promote" chemotherapy since "it was demonstrated" that it had "proved to be an effective treatment for cancer patients, not only in the United States, but around the world."[1]

In the years that followed, many scientists, doctors and cancer patients were encouraged with the hope that very soon a cure would be found for cancer.

Then came the official declaration of war on cancer. In December 1971, in cooperation with the American Cancer Society (ACS), President Richard M. Nixon signed the National Cancer Act. With it came the promise of a victory over cancer and a 50 percent reduction of the cancer death rate in ten years, if sufficient funds were provided.[2]

Perhaps this would be the initiative that would win the battle against cancer. With all these forces brought together, maybe it was the time for an answer.

But five years later, in an annual assembly, the directors of the President's Cancer Panel reported that no positive results could be shown, no progress had been made.[3] Then in 1980 the NCI felt obliged to report that very little ground had been gained, and its members were fearful of a loss of prestige.[4]

In fact, despite modern technology, research and an abundance of funds, cancer deaths were up. In 1972 about 330,000 patients died of cancer in the United States. Despite the promise to cut that figure in half in a decade, by 1982 the cancer death rate surpassed the 400,000 mark.[5]

In 1984, under Dr. Vincent T. De Vita, the NCI theatrically announced the "reachable" goal of reducing the death rate by 50 percent in twenty years (1980–2000). That meant that since 490,000 people died of cancer in 1980, only 245,000 people would die of cancer at the beginning of the twenty-first century.[6]

The Hope of Living Cancer Free

LOSING THE WAR

WE ARE LOSING the war. The advances against cancer—in surgery, radiation and chemotherapy—have left much to be desired in view of the fact that the most common forms of cancer remain uncontrollable. In May 1986, Dr. John C. Bailar III of Harvard University and Elaine Smith of the University of Iowa published in the New England Journal of Medicine an "atomic bomb" against orthodox oncology. Bailar and Smith insisted that the scientific world reconsider the current guiding principles of cancer research, along with their application.

The death rate of cancer patients continued to rise in comparison to cardiovascular diseases, where a downward trend in the death rate was evident. Dr. Bailar and his team concluded that they "were losing the war against cancer," and that "substantial progress in the understanding of the nature and attributes of cancer" had not led to "a reduction of the incidence of mortality." Therefore, they asserted that "the most promising areas of cancer research are those of prevention rather than treatment."[7]

In spite of the prestige of these authors and their respective universities and the strength of their argument, their wise recommendations went in one ear and out the other as far as the scientific community was concerned. At the start of the twenty-first century, billions of dollars and twenty-nine years after Nixon's declaration of war on cancer, the outlook for the effective treatment of cancer is still discouraging.[8]

Let's compare this prediction with what is occurring. In 1985 over 485,000 people died from cancer.[9] In 1995 the ACS predicted 525,000 deaths, but some statisticians concluded the actual number was close to 700,000.[10]

A depressing picture of the effectiveness of "approved" treatments against cancer (surgery, radiation and chemotherapy) was revealed in an evaluation made by the ACS in 1996. Their annual publication of *Cancer Facts and Figures* shows virtually no improvement in the death rates among those with the most frequently appearing tumors in the last sixty years, with the exception of cancer of the stomach and cervix.

The improvement in the death rates for people suffering from cancer of the stomach is an enigma since the conventional treatments have not been successful. The improvements are most likely due to better hygiene, healthier foods and the advent of endoscopy, which detects gastric diseases in the early stages. However, the treatments themselves for this type of cancer—surgery, chemotherapy and radiation—have not been shown to contribute to the improvement in the mortality rate.

The approved treatment for cervical-uterine cancer—again, surgery, chemotherapy and radiation—is likewise not responsible for the improvement in the death rate in that category. In fact, the downward slope in the graph indicates that improvement began a long time before modern scientific advances, such as radiation therapy, were introduced.

The Pap smear has drastically reduced cervical-uterine cancer deaths. It is the invention of a simple test by Dr. George Papanicolaou in 1928 (now named after him) that detects cervical cancer.

The "enormous scientific advances" have not helped patients survive. On the contrary, where the malignancies, such as cancer of the lung and breast, are treated with aggressive remedies (surgery, chemotherapy and radiation), the death rates are incredibly high.[11]

The death rate of people suffering from pulmonary cancer has literally exploded. Since 1960 there has been an increase in death rate by lung cancer in women. I assume this is due to the fact that many women began smoking cigarettes in the 1960s during the Women's Liberation Movement. For reasons unknown, women seem more susceptible than men to the harmful effects of cigarette smoke,[12] and they are consequently more susceptible to lung cancer. Now lung cancer is the number one cancer killer in women, the same as in men![13] I'm sure this was not the equality women were searching for.

WHERE ARE THE VICTORIES?

THE TECHNOLOGICAL REVOLUTION has created impressive new products in almost every branch of industry. Today, no one would buy a ten-year-old computer; in America, even a six-month-old computer is virtually outdated!

Most branches of medicine have also seen significant technological changes. For example, plastic catheters are now so sophisticated that they can remain inside the body for years. The old ones that could only be left in place for a few weeks have been abandoned.

However, in the treatment of cancer, no substantial improvement has occurred. The medical community continues to fight cancer with the same weapons as before—surgery, radiation and chemotherapy—only more sophisticated versions. However, they have not produced any better results for the cancer victim.

What about the field of genetics? In 1994 the cover of the April 25 edition of *Time* magazine proclaimed that "new discoveries promise improved therapies and hope in the war against cancer." The article referred to discoveries related to genetic mutations associated with the formation of specific tumors. Unfortunately, the therapeutic application of these discoveries remains in the far distant future.

Scientists have been working in these areas since the 1960s, and their results are still minimal. Plus, in manipulating genes, scientists are delving into the heart of creation. The risks are enormous, and the consequences might be worse than the diseases.

Since the United States' sponsoring of the Genome Project, the genetic mapping of the human body, gene business has exploded in spite of the tremendous social fears it engenders. People have always wanted to know the future, but not necessarily how they are going to die.

Insurance companies would be seriously interested in such formidable cost-effective information, especially if they could find out the genetic burden of a child before he or she is born. Since rising medical costs have forced many companies into bankruptcy, employers could minimize the risk by disposing of genetically challenged employees.[14]

Geneticists argue that privacy laws and governmental policies can address societal concerns. The potential for benefits in diagnosis, coupled with the enormous future in the genetic capabilities to produce human spare parts, could change the medical practice 180 degrees. But the gains of genetic science could allow people to come up with a desirable genetic blueprint, which brings to mind oppression of the weak. All this is a plausible future.

A QUALIFIED FAILURE

SO IF WE are losing our war on cancer, it makes sense to look for an alternative battle plan. In other branches of modern science and industry, new and improved processes continually replace the old ones—even if the old ones still work. Things have to improve!

But regarding the cancer issue, science continues to beat the same dead horse. Courses of treatment that have shown poor results are still being used. Governmental authorities, the scientific community and pharmaceutical companies seem to want to continue to use drugs, including chemotherapy drugs, that have been shown to be ineffective. Perhaps one reason is that developing a new drug is a very expensive process. Getting a medication through clinical trials and FDA approval costs millions of dollars.

We can understand the cost of prescription drugs when we consider how much money the manufacturer spends just on the approval process. Plus, it spends money on research and development and marketing. So it is easy to see the need to market approved medications in order to recoup the initial investment. Plus, we can see how pharmaceutical companies might not want people to discover that they could do without drugs by changing their eating habits and lifestyles. Illness and disease are big business!

But the evidence is mounting that these pharmaceuticals are not working as planned. In fact, it is well known that patients suffering from many malignancies live longer and better if the orthodox treatments (surgery, radiation and chemotherapy) are not applied.

In 1969, Dr. Hardin James of the University of California at Berkeley reported at an ACS conference that patients not subjected to the aggressive conventional therapies actually had a *longer* life expectancy than those who were, occasionally up to four times as long. Drs. Bailar and Smith, in the 1986 *New England Journal of Medicine* article already mentioned, reported along the same lines. They noted that patients with lung cancer who were *not* treated had a longer life expectancy and enjoyed a better quality of life than those who received treatment.[15]

Bailar, upon evaluating the results of cancer therapies done between 1950 and 1980, rated them to be a "qualified failure."[16]

In an experiment with patients suffering from pancreatic cancer, those who received the placebo treatment instead of the real treatment lived longer and better, reported Dr. Ulrich Abel, Ph.D., of the University of Heidelberg, in 1988.[17]

It seems like common sense, in the face of these "qualified" testimonies, to conclude that more doctors should avoid conventional treatment or prescribe placebos. But most doctors aren't used to prescribing no treatment at all. Plus, pharmaceutical companies urge doctors to use their products, for obvious reasons. And, prescribing placebos or no treatment at all outside the confines of an experimental setting may present to the doctor an ethical dilemma.

THE CURRENT STATISTICS

A GOOD WAY to see how goes the battle is to look at the cancer facts and figures. The information available at the American Cancer Society's Internet site (www.cancer.org) is vast. A chart of the American Cancer Society's projection of deaths and incidences of all cancers by site for just the year of 1999 can be found in Appendix A.

Although the figures on this chart are conservative, still 1,221,800 people were expected to get cancer for the first time in 1999. That is one half of 1 percent of the total population of the United States. The chart also shows that 563,100 people will die in 1999 from cancer. That means 1,500 Americans are dying from cancer every single day.

According to the American Cancer Society, 8.2 million Americans currently have cancer.[18] That is 3 percent of the total population. Now 3 percent may not sound like much, but think about it. If you go to a church with one hundred members, the statistics suggest that three of those people have cancer, whether you know who they are or not. If you go to a movie theater that seats two hundred people, six people there with you are battling for their lives. What if you attend the Rose Bowl, the first one of the new millennium, on January 1, 2000? It seats roughly one hundred thousand people. You wouldn't know who they were, but three thousand of those people, no matter which team they cheered for, would have cancer.

Cancer deaths are second only to those related to heart

disease,[19] but cancer will surely overtake the lead in this dreaded category during the first decade of the twenty-first century.

IT'S TIME FOR
ALTERNATIVE THERAPIES

IT SEEMS OBVIOUS that current treatment methods and the direction of cancer research must change. For decades we have been barking up the wrong tree, and the public is getting wise to this.

Pasteur's quest to conquer the germ reminds us that the medical system today is based on pharmaceuticals. Doctors are trained to prescribe medication for most illnesses, and pharmaceutical companies do a good job selling doctors on their new products. This is not news to you. Many patients have left their doctors' offices with prescriptions in hand, but no satisfaction that their maladies were treated or their complaints were even heard.

Based on all this, it shouldn't surprise us that the established system is not open to new and alternative therapies. There is no place for them in it. Though many alternative therapies have been proven effective and do not deteriorate the patients' quality of life, they are ridiculed, pushed aside and prohibited by the medical establishment. *Yet patients are demanding them.*[20]

Although I have seen wonderful advances in the alternative medical world, I have not seen any therapy that consistently produces remissions in every patient with every type of cancer. I am a strong believer and promoter of natural, nontoxic and noninvasive therapies, but I am aware of their limitations as well. It may surprise you that I don't believe that we can put our hope in medical research—*conventional or alternative*.

Hope for a Cure

After watching the scientific community spend exorbitant amounts of money on decades of unsuccessful research to find a cure for cancer, I have come to a new conclusion regarding our fight against cancer: *Prevention is the best medicine.* But more on that later.

For now, it is easy to understand why cancer is so feared. The statistics are getting worse instead of better, no matter how much money we throw at the problem. We can see why cancer has been regarded as a death sentence. People with cancer face a tough dilemma: to fight the disease when the available therapies promise little help, or to fly from the problem and say, "It doesn't matter what I do, so *que sera, sera.*"

Given all this, it is easy to feel hopeless, as if we are fighting against the odds. Cancer seems to have the upper hand no matter what we do. Is there truly any hope?

TAKE CONTROL

I HAVE SEEN so many people beat the odds. Most of the victors have had positive mental attitudes. Even the pessimists who beat the odds have had positive people around them—wives or husbands, mothers or friends who remained optimistic and encouraging.

If you have cancer, I encourage you to tackle the problem head-on and decide that, no matter what happens, cancer won't triumph over you emotionally. If we just give up, cancer has won the ultimate battle—the one fought over the human spirit, not the body. If we fight with a passion that will not give up against any odds, we can turn the tables on cancer.

My goal is to motivate you to think for yourself and investigate for yourself. Find out what you can before you need to know it. Many universities let the public into their medical libraries, and there you can study the reports on different therapies in the medical journals. If you are facing a treatment decision today, get two or three opinions. You are in charge, and the treatment you feel the most positive about is the one you should choose.

We need to change our thinking about cancer. The status quo just doesn't work. Modern therapies are ineffective and even harmful. New ideas, new ways of thinking and a new humility will bring breakthroughs and hope.

Now, let's explore the causes of cancer and what therapies exist to treat it.

Section II:
Restoration From Within

5

Restoring the Inner Man

WHAT WOULD HAPPEN if a general told his soldiers on the eve of a great battle that, statistically speaking, 90 percent of them would die? As they prepare for battle, the general shouts, "This is a lost cause—in the end you will have died for nothing!"

Cancer specialists often assault hope—by delivering the harsh clinical statistics of death with a cold certainty, for fear of offending the "honesty" of our profession (and the lawyers).

In some cultures, a cancer diagnosis is kept from the patient. While I do not recommend that extreme, I also do not believe bad news has to be delivered in an antiseptic, statistical manner.

When we doctors deliver a diagnosis of cancer with professional certainty, the patient goes home and prepares to die—not to fight. That's because the great missing ingredient in this verdict is hope. Hope does not abound in cancer circles, especially in oncological centers. In fact, hopelessness in the face of a horrendous death is the scourge of cancer.

Many patients are internally conditioned to submit meekly to such terrible decrees. After all, a doctor gave the sentence, and what he says is law. If an oncologist tells a patient that he has only three months to live, the patient will be anxiously waiting to fall dead on that prescribed day.

Why am I making such a fuss about this? Because our emotions and mental attitudes not only affect our immune system, but they also actually *determine* its response. Our ability to fight cancer—or to avoid getting it in the first place—depends on how we react in the face of adversity. A key element of hope for living cancer free is restoring, undergirding and strengthening the inner man: our minds, hearts, wills and emotions.

THE IMPACT OF STRESS
ON THE IMMUNE SYSTEM

STRESS SEEMS TO be an integral part of modern life. It presses in upon us from everywhere—our jobs, our families, our neighbors, other drivers, the weather—you name it. You may think that these stresses create our attitudes, and they can. But it also works the other way around: Our internal attitudes impact our bodies. What you think, feel and believe can determine your health.

The immune system—this complex, sophisticated defender of the human race—is deeply affected by our internal attitudes, emotions and spiritual fortitude.

I define stress as "a deficit of resources needed to resolve a problem." This is a simple but adequate definition. If you have enough money to pay the rent, there is no stress; when you hear the footsteps of the landlord, however, and you have to give him an excuse, anxiety reigns! The lack of resources stresses us.

Good mental health promotes good physical health, according to George Lilans, a Boston psychiatrist. He followed the lives of two hundred Harvard graduates for thirty years and studied data from medical examinations and psychological tests. Lilans discovered a clear link between unhappiness and disease or death.

Many of my own patients can point to stressful situations they feel helped to trigger their cancer. But how can you measure the impact our emotions have on the immune system? The following is a scale created by Dr. Thomas H. Holmes and Dr. Richard H. Rehi of the University of Washington Medical School that measures each stress situation with a point system.[1]

Death of a spouse 100

Divorce 73

Separation from a spouse 65

Imprisonment 63

Death of a family member 63

Sickness or accident 53

Marriage 50

Stopping work 47

Reconciliation in marriage 45

Retirement procedures 45

Family illness 44

Pregnancy 40

Sexual problems 39

A new person in the family 39

Personal readjustment 39

Financial adjustment 38

Death of a friend 37

Job change 36

Family discussions 35

Mortgages above $25,000 31

Debt foreclosure 30

Heavier responsibilities 29

Children leaving home 29

Wife starting work 26

Beginning or ending classes 26
Change of residence 25
Change of personal habits 24
Problems with the boss 23
Change of work hours 20
Change of neighborhood 20
Change of school 20
Change of recreation 19
Change of church 19
Change of social activities 18
Small mortgage 18
Change of sleeping habits 16
Separation from family 15
Change of diet 15
Planning a vacation 13
Christmas activities 12
Misdemeanors 11

Holmes and his collaborators were actually able to predict illnesses on the basis of this scale. Almost half (49 percent) of the people who had accumulated three hundred points in a twelve-month period developed some critical illness, while only 9 percent of those who accumulated less than two hundred points in the same period fell ill. This experiment irrefutably establishes the impact that accumulated stress can have on our bodies.

Some people who have a greater capacity for managing stress are less susceptible to falling ill. Additionally, losing one's job at age twenty-five is not the same as losing it at fifty, nor is it the same to end a marriage by common consent as it is to end it in the midst of a heated battle.

Happy, positive events as well as sad, problematic ones can cause stress. Getting married, for example, means joining with a beloved person—it is a happy event. Even so, it implies an adaptation that requires effort on the part of both parties, so it can be stressful.

Either way, bear in mind that our emotions determine the response of our immune system. Why do some fall ill under stressful situations while others do not? It depends on how we react to the stressor.

In order to grasp this fully, let's look at the immune system itself. It is your own personal militia, patrolling for enemy invaders and destroying them. And it awaits your (unconscious) command. I would like to help you understand as well as possible (and don't think your doctor completely understands it) what your body counts on to maintain health. Come with me on an abbreviated tour.

THE IMMUNE SYSTEM

THE MASTER WORK of creation is the human being, but with all the splendor and greatness that God gave us, our survival is still very fragile. In a world plagued by invisible aggressors, the importance of our defense mechanisms looms large. Although the body relies on some natural barriers like the skin, nasal hair, mucus secretions and inflammatory processes, the bulk of the defense task falls on the immune system.

The moment a microorganism enters the body, an elaborate and extremely intricate attack is launched. The capillaries dilate like flexible tunnels to admit an army of defenders called leukocytes. Like all truly efficient lines of defense, the immune system attacks with a strategy that is divided initially into two types of responses: the nonspecific and the specific.

The nonspecific immune response

The nonspecific immune response is the main system of defense for newborns until they develop antibodies. However, this response never ceases to be useful and necessary. Tribes of white corpuscles called monocytes and phagocytes are charged with attacking any invader never before encountered.

Macrophages are derived from the monocytes. Present in almost all organic tissue, they have the mission of surrounding and disintegrating undesirable cells. From the phagocytes come microphages, which are divided into two sections—the neutrophils and the eosinophils. The neutrophils are a large army in charge of disintegrating invading bacteria. The eosinophils, a more select group, target foreign substances such as cells covered by antibodies and allergens.

The specific immune response

After birth the specific immune response develops as a response to microorganisms and their toxins. This gigantic task can only be accomplished by the awesome lymphocytes, so called because they are produced by lymphatic ganglia. One-fourth of all white cells are lymphocytes, which are divided into three branches—T cells, B cells and NK cells (natural killer). These are distributed strategically according to specific needs throughout the body.

The T cells are cytotoxic. In other words, they poison the invaders through chemical warfare. This is such an important line of defense that 80 percent of the lymphocytes are T cells. Another 15 percent of the lymphocytes are B cells. These are more specialized, producing the mighty immunoglobulins, which are exceedingly important antibodies. In a process we call humoral immunity, immunoglobulins maintain the memory of which specific chemical substances will destroy a specific invader. The killer cells, the remaining 5 percent, are the SWAT team of the lymphocytes. With brute force they charge invaders or aberrant cells like cancer or cells infected with a virus.

The immune system in action

So then, the leukocytes (white blood cells) in all their branches are the assault troops that attack when outside invaders put the body in danger. Invisible slippery fighters loaded with weapons, they maneuver around the cells, good and bad, like Tijuana taxi drivers on a busy boulevard, confronting pathogenic microorganisms face to face.

Seen through a microscope, the lymphocytes look like over-easy eggs sprinkled with ground pepper. Each "little dot of pepper" is a deadly chemical weapon. The neutrophils in the bloodstream inflate themselves like balloons before they attack. The microphages just seem to lie around, buried among the tissues, but they spring to life when there is an attack. The neutrophils, armed with proteins and nonspecific chemical agents, do the job of common soldiers, attacking the enemy with brute force and a numerical advantage.

Lymphocytes, like combat tanks, arrive with the heavy artillery. Their strategy may vary. While some lymphocytes float in the blood and attack any foreign microorganisms that travel along, others plant themselves in vital organs and pursue any invaders that may have gotten past the first line of defense. Still other lymphocytes corral the invaders in the lymph nodes, which serve as execution chambers.

When the battle is over, the neutrophils gather up cellular refuse and perform a vital clean-up job. Because pathogens can camouflage themselves with chemical barriers made up of cellular refuse, cytoplasmic seepage, coagulating agents and destroyed membranes, the clean-up crews are led by the antibodies, which guide the lymphocytes to the camouflaged pathogens. Although the antibodies are one thousand times smaller than bacteria, they attach themselves to their enemy like *banderillas* attached to a bull in a bullfight, weakening and neutralizing its irregular forms in preparation for the definitive attack by the *matadors,* the leukocytes.

The Hope of Living Cancer Free

In healthy periods, twenty-five billion leukocytes circulate freely in the bloodstream, and another twenty-five billion rest on the walls of the blood vessels and other tissues. When an infection appears, billions of reserves leap into the bloodstream from the bone marrow. The blood can quickly mobilize up to ten times the normal number of leukocytes. Doctors can therefore measure the seriousness of an infection by the number of leukocytes in the blood. The higher the number, the greater the degree of virulence.

The first time an agent invades the body, one of the circulating lymphocytes (B cells) comes in contact with this pathogen, memorizes its shape and size and dashes to the nearest lymph node. This lymphocyte then turns into a chemical factory, transferring the recently acquired information to thousands of other lymphocytes. All these lymphocytes become factories that produce antibodies. In a few hours the body will have billions of antibodies specifically designed to kill the new invaders. Once the lymph nodes produce an antibody, the formula remains stored permanently so that when the aggression is again present, the response can be immediate.

The antibodies are the highest expressions of specific immunity. An antibody protects our organism from a single affliction. For example, the antibody against the measles virus has no effect on the smallpox virus.

The timing of the immune response is a greater determiner of success than is the response itself. The body needs time to organize its defenses. Here antibiotics shine because they destroy millions of bacteria, giving the body that crucial time. But an antibiotic never kills all the germs. Even if it kills all but one, that lone microbe can immediately reproduce itself in industrial quantities. Only the immune system does away with 100 percent of the invaders.

But even with these setbacks, we can't deny that the

human race has survived all these centuries, thanks to the immune system.

THE POWER OF THE NEGATIVE

ARNOLD HUTSCHNECKER, AUTHOR of *The Will to Live,* wrote, "Depression is a partial surrender to death, and it seems that cancer is desperation at the cellular level."[2]

Humans are obsessed with the negative. Have you ever seen a TV news broadcaster who gives only good news? I heard an unusual individual who tried that and promptly went bankrupt. Stress is bad for you, and it is often a contributing cause for disease.

Much of the early work demonstrating that emotions can cause illness was undertaken by Hans Seyle at the University of Prague in the 1920s.[3] Later as a director of the Institute of Experimental Medicine and Surgery at the University of Montreal, Seyle "discovered that chronic stress suppresses the immune system which is responsible for engulfing and destroying cancerous cells or alien microorganisms. The important point is this: The physical conditions Seyle describes as being produced by stress are virtually identical to those under which abnormal cells could reproduce and spread into dangerous cancer."[4]

In the modern world we are under constant emotional pressure. Crises and wars are everywhere. How can we avoid the stress that anguish, fear and depression cause?

The actions and reactions of our bodies are, more than anything else, responses to the attitudes with which we confront the events, problems, challenges, experiences, memories and expectations of our lives. Researchers are just discovering how depression, pessimism, excitement and optimism directly and physically affect the reactions and capabilities of our immune system. Yet Galen, in the second century, had already asserted that depressed men or women

more easily fell prey to cancer than those of a more san-
guine temperament.

Evidence published by Dr. William Morton of the
University of Oregon shows that stay-at-home-moms who
feel useless contract cancer with 54 percent more frequency
than the general population and with a 157 percent higher
incidence than women who work.[5] Wives and mothers who
feel they make a substantial contribution, who know they
are an irreplaceable team member in the family, have a
lower incidence of cancer. What an awesome correlation
between frustration and dissatisfaction and the crippling of
the body's system of defense.

Divorced persons have the highest index of cardiovascular
disease, pneumonia, high blood pressure, cancer and, even
though you may doubt it, fatal accidents (camouflaged sui-
cides?). Did you notice on the stress scale that divorce causes
more stress than imprisonment? The number of couples split-
ting up because of irreconcilable differences is staggering. A
lot of people out there are in high-risk categories.

We have a society of depressed, resentful adults and of children who either hate themselves because they feel responsible
for a divorce or hate their parents because they were abandoned by them. It shouldn't surprise us that *Time* magazine
stated, "The history of hate in the family is one of the primary
factors which determines risk, the risk of contracting cancer,
the most devastating plague of the twentieth century."[6]

THE POWER OF THE POSITIVE

UNTIL VERY RECENTLY, giving hope to patients was considered
almost criminal. We have chosen "Oasis of Hope" as the
name of our Contreras Cancer Care Center because our
whole existence depends on hope.

After I delivered a speech in an oncological meeting
recently, a colleague accused me of selling "false" hope.

Trying to calm him down, I asked him what his definition of "true" hope was. I intended the question to help him understand that either there is hope, or there is not. Hope is not true or false. To hope or not to hope—this is what the patient faces. Doctors fear encouraging their patients' hope, because they know the limitations of the available therapies. Yet hopelessness makes cancer the victor.

Thank God, more and more doctors are acknowledging the value of encouraging their patients. But love for the patient was exchanged long ago for the academic passion for research. Feelings, emotions, fears and expectations are still ridiculed. This is tragic, especially in view of scientific research that shows how much a patient benefits from a hopeful perspective.

The happy person is not the one who has only good things happen to him or her, but is the one who keeps a positive attitude, even in adverse circumstances. A great part of this positive attitude is spiritual. Those who can rest in God, trusting Him no matter what, do better in difficult situations.

In the Bible we read of the prophet Habakkuk, who in the midst of good times cried out:

> Although the fig tree shall not blossom, neither shall fruit be in the vines; the labour of the olive shall fail, and the fields shall yield no meat; the flock shall be cut off from the fold, and there shall be no herd in the stalls: Yet I will rejoice in the LORD, I will joy in the God of my salvation. The LORD God is my strength, and he will make my feet like hinds' feet, and he will make me to walk upon mine high places.
>
> —HABAKKUK 3:17–19

Habakkuk was ready and willing to keep a positive outlook, giving thanks even if his fate would turn for the worst.

The concept that we are children of an almighty God who

cares about us and acts on behalf of our problems is mythical for most. God is a concept, not a being, to most—much less a person of action. But Jesus said:

> Which of you, if his son asks for bread, will give him a stone? Or if he asks for a fish, will give him a snake? If you, then, though you are evil, know how to give good gifts to your children, how much more will your Father in heaven give good gifts to those who ask him!
> —MATTHEW 7:9–11, NIV

If science convinces you that it is not reasonable to believe in a loving God, then you cannot take advantage of the huge benefits—physical and spiritual—that faith provides.

But if you embrace the offer of trusting in God's care for you, and you earnestly and reasonably put your trust in God, your perceptions about life and its problems begin to shift. The action of God is often suffocated and strangulated when we don't give it all over to Him.

I often counsel my patients to turn their fear of the cancer that is attacking their bodies over to God. I have watched as these individuals are relieved of their fear and respond better to the treatments. It is almost as if cancer has a mind of its own and thinks, *It is no fun attacking this person; he isn't afraid of me anymore.* And the cancer leaves that person's body and looks for another victim.

What really happens is that the stress caused by fear is detrimental to the immune system. A person with a depressed immune system has a much harder time fighting off cancer. When a person can release the fear, the stress is reduced, and the immune system will function better to help the patient win the battle against cancer.

In all these things we can reach for the highest and best. Let's cultivate the habit of thinking big, and we will learn to use words that will allow God to make us conquerors. Let's not say we can't when God has said He can.

ATTITUDES: MESSAGES TO OUR BODIES

POSITIVE OR NEGATIVE attitudes act as messages from our minds, conscious or unconscious, that are capable of engaging biochemical processes in our organisms that directly affect the state of alert of our immune system. Body functions, from an insignificant muscle twitch to the amount of white cells circulating, are all dependent on our state of mind. They are activated or blocked by biochemical messages, probably through enzymes or hormones like the endorphins.

It is important to give our bodies the right messages through our attitudes. We do not want to give them negative messages—or mixed messages.

A cancer patient from Chicago who had been told to settle his affairs and get ready to die came to see me. I asked him why an affluent stockbroker such as himself would choose to come to a retrograde country—and of all places, Tijuana—to seek help from a supposed quack.

"Because you are the only one who offers me some ray of hope," was his telling reply. This man was willing to cross frontiers, not only geographical but also cultural, to demonstrate that he was committed to regain his body's health.

"What do you have in your shirt pocket?" I asked him.

"It's a pack of cigarettes."

"Sir, you have lung cancer. Don't you think it would be a good idea to stop smoking?"

"Yes, I definitely know that is what I ought to do, but I haven't been able to stop."

Here is a clear example of mixed messages. On the one hand, the patient is saying to his body, "I am so interested in you that I am willing to travel to Mexico. I have been given up on, but I will try alternative medicine. I want to go on living." On the other hand, by refusing to quit smoking, the patient is saying to his body, "My commitment does not include doing away with the pleasure of smoking, even though cigarettes are killing you."

The healing process requires that the patient be 100 percent committed to getting well. Our bodies are too clever for anything less.

Getting well—what does it take? Many factors are involved, yes, but it all boils down to the impact each one of those factors has on the immune system. And of all the factors, the greatest of these is love.

THE POWER OF LOVE

NO DRUG ON the market even comes close to producing the positive effects of love. If scientists could find a way to encapsulate love, they would have the marketing dream of the century—the breakthrough of the millennium. The cost would be low, and the side effects would be welcomed!

Although love research is in its infancy, studies are beginning to confirm its positive effects. The Menninger Foundation of Topeka, Kansas, found that people in love had lower levels of lactic acid in the bloodstream, which caused them to feel less tired. They also had higher levels of endorphins, which caused them to feel more euphoric and less sensitive to pain. Their white corpuscles responded better to infection, and they caught fewer colds.[7]

A most revealing work was done in Israel by Jack Medalie and Uri Goldbourt.[8] The two researchers studied ten thousand men with high-risk conditions such as angina pectoris, anxiety, high cholesterol and irregular heartbeat—all precursors of a fatal cardiovascular condition. Through psychological testing they determined with a high degree of certainty who would have a heart attack and who would not.

After all was said and done, the ones who had the highest

incidence of heart attacks were the ones who answered no to the question, "Does your wife show you love?"[9]

Life insurance companies have discovered that men who leave for work in the morning with a kiss from their wives are better clients because they will have fewer car accidents and will, on the average, live five years longer.[10] If insurance companies weren't in the business of evaluating risk to increase their revenue, I wouldn't believe it either. But there it is—simple and romantically scientific!

In 1982 Harvard psychologists David McClelland and Carol Tishnit discovered that even films about love increase human levels of immunoglobulin-A in saliva, the first line of defense against colds and other viral diseases. Although this immunological improvement lasted less than an hour, it could be prolonged by having the subjects think about moments in their lives when someone loved them.[11] If we love, we are happy; those around us make up a part of our positive world and don't wear down our defenses.

I welcome research on love. Perhaps when its value is proven, doctors will take advantage of this powerful knowledge in their daily practice.

It is not surprising that the essence of the biblical message is love, immortally described by St. Paul:

> Though I speak with the tongues of men and of angels, but have not love, I have become as sounding brass or a clanging cymbal. And though I have the gift of prophecy, and understand all mysteries and all knowledge, and though I have all faith, so that I could remove mountains, but have not love, I am nothing. And though I bestow all my goods to feed the poor, and though I give my body to be burned, but have not love, it profits me nothing.
>
> Love suffers long and is kind; love does not envy; love

does not parade itself, is not puffed up; does not behave rudely, does not seek its own, is not provoked, thinks no evil; does not rejoice in iniquity, but rejoices in the truth; bears all things, believes all things, hopes all things, endures all things.

Love never fails. But whether there are prophecies, they will fail; whether there are tongues, they will cease; whether there is knowledge, it will vanish away....And now abide faith, hope, love, these three; but the greatest of these is love.

—1 CORINTHIANS 13:1–8, 13, NKJV

ATTITUDE RULES

STORIES OF TWO of my patients exemplify the dramatic power of love and hope—or the lack of it. A nineteen-year-old woman who had been diagnosed with cancer of the small intestine came in to see me in late 1975. The course of chemotherapy she had already been given offered no positive results. Under these conditions, her prognosis was death within three to six months. Her doctors had given up hope.

This girl was a member of her country's team, which in eight months was participating in the Olympic games in Montreal. She came to me because she did not accept the prognosis of her doctors, and she told me that under no circumstances would she miss the competition.

As you can imagine, she began her treatment with a lot of faith and discipline. The results were indeed amazing. In all truth, our results with patients with this type of tumor are poor. But her determination and tenacity stimulated her defenses so powerfully that they destroyed her tumor.

I believe the treatment only served as an emotional reinforcement. All she needed was somebody to give her hope, somebody to show interest and love. As of the writing of this book, this patient is alive and healthy.

I also remember a middle-aged woman with breast cancer who came to me after having had her left breast removed. Her cancer had metastasized into her bones and lungs. Conventional therapies had failed, and her doctors sent her home to die.

At the start of our treatment, the remains of her former beauty could only be faintly seen. She looked like a skeleton, and she was bald. All of this was the result of aggressive and unsuccessful treatment with chemotherapy.

Little by little she began to improve. Her hair grew back, she gained weight and the beauty of her face reappeared. In six months, she was a new person. Although surgical mutilation had dealt her a painful blow, she overcame it.

Once her husband saw that she was strong enough to deal with it, he asked her for a divorce. This is devastating event under any circumstances, but in this case she interpreted it as a rejection of her mutilated body. Within three weeks, she experienced an explosion of tumors.

Although she came back to see me, she confessed that the loss of her husband's love represented the worst kind of rejection to her. Life had lost all meaning. No human power was able to change her perspective. Her immune system gave up, and the tumors took advantage of the open doors and killed her.

How to Love Ourselves the Right Way

LOVE IS SO important and powerful that Christ summarized all the commandments into one, the Golden Rule: "Love your neighbor as you love yourself." But why is there so little love? My brother-in-law, Joel Ordaz, an independent minister, says our problems are precisely *because* we love our neighbors as we love ourselves!

So, how do we love ourselves? We do it by eating junk food, drinking alcoholic beverages and smoking. Love is never having to exercise. We love ourselves by quarreling, fighting and having to get our way. Our neighbors certainly don't need to be loved with that kind of love!

Self-esteem in every culture is vital to the preservation of good health, both physical and mental. Narcissists love just their looks, but people who love or esteem themselves accept the fact that they are imperfect beings. Once you and your defects are comfortable with each other, you are more likely to be happy in this world. Those who are at peace with themselves and others enjoy a longer and better life.

This love of self includes accepting responsibility for the health of your body, soul and spirit. Even with our imperfections, love is still the answer.

BEING LOVED BY GOD

EACH OF US is designed to be a unified creature—body, soul and spirit. Though the pace of modern life doesn't leave room to cultivate a whole and balanced life, we cannot be divided. Those who give exclusive importance to the body but neglect intellect and the spirit are failing to practice adequate medicine.

The cultivation of the spirit is putting meaningful time into our relationship with God. The spirit is that part of our being that allows us to communicate with God. It is what allows hopeless human beings to recover the essence of life in a supernatural way, to discover life as never before.

Every person who has spiritual ties—no matter his or her religious beliefs—lives longer and better. But the great advantage of Christianity is that it is founded on love.

> For God so loved the world, that he gave his only begotten Son, that whosoever believeth in him should not perish, but have everlasting life.
>
> —JOHN 3:16

This manifestation of the love of God to mankind is what enables us to love ourselves and others. It also is the foundation of hope that whatever we do is not in vain, that we are going to a special eternal place where there will be no more sorrow or pain.

To see the human person as a trinity—body, mind and spirit—and then to treat him as such in the practice of medicine is something I learned from my father. When I chat with my patients, I make sure they leave with useful hope that can help them confront their condition.

We can see that many factors can affect the status of our immune system—fear, stress, attitude, hope, love and trust in God. Now let's look at the external factors that can affect our health and lead to cancer.

6

Restoring the Body

THE TRADITIONAL GOAL of cancer research has been to find cancer-killing agents. But if I were going to look for the cure to cancer, I would focus on identifying what causes cancer.

The common denominator in cause of cancer—or any chronic degenerative disease—is stress put on the body that breaks down the harmony the body needs to function correctly. Stress, both external and internal, breaks the balance by tearing down our immune defense system and increasing our susceptibility to cancer.

Internal stressors are things that happen in our mental, emotional and spiritual lives. Most people think of stress as emotional or psychological: Too much to do, a family crisis or pressure from the boss makes us *feel* stressed. In the last chapter we learned that since stress can manifest itself in physical illnesses, managing emotional and spiritual stress is critical. Now, let's take a look at the stress on our immune systems coming from our external environment. Hope for living cancer free includes restoring the body from the devastating affects of a toxic environment.

The Hope of Living Cancer Free

Not only can we be stressed emotionally, but our bodies can also be stressed physically. If we're in the desert, over-heated and without water, we're experiencing physical stress. Architects and engineers who design buildings look at the structure to make sure it can handle the stress on it from the weight and pressure of the building materials.

In this same way, physical illness can be the result of external stress. We come into daily contact with the causes of physical stress. Let's see what some of them are.

CONTAMINATION OF THE WATER SUPPLY

THE HUMAN RACE has always used the ocean and other bodies of water as giant natural trash cans, believing that the various biological cycles would absorb the waste and purify the water. Though the water cycle was designed to do just that, it was not designed to handle the synthetic waste or the quantity of contaminants being dumped into our waters.

The advent of the petrochemical industry in this century led to the manufacture of synthetic products—some that cost less than before and others that were totally new useful items that thrilled consumers. In that year one billion pounds of synthetic chemical substances were produced. Production increased to fifty billion pounds in the following decade, and by the 1980s, production exceeded half a trillion pounds. Would nature be able to deal with all of these chemicals?

In the United States, there are four million recognized chemical compounds. This number increases each year by approximately one thousand new compounds. The time and cost of laboratory tests for carcinogenesis, teratogenesis and so on makes it impossible to keep up with production. Millions of substances have not been tested for safety at all, yet it is known that some six hundred of them are highly carcinogenic (cancer-causing).

It took three decades and millions of dollars to unequivo-

cally prove that tobacco causes cancer. The producers of cigarettes relied on huge economic resources to counteract these
investigations. Just imagine the vast resources of the petrochemical industry! Meanwhile, these chemicals and their
by-products are spoiling the soil and the water.

Unfortunately, water treatment plants cannot even detect,
much less detoxify, most of the chemical substances dumped
into the water. Present methods of treatment consist of fil-
tering out dangerous waste from known sources of
contaminants. This is a good start, but the reality is that new
contaminants escape even the most modern filtration systems.

Toxic Waste

In May 1971, at the Shenandoah Stables in St. Louis, thirty-
eight hundred liters of oil were spread on the ground to
control the dust stirred up in the arena where the horses
were trained—a common practice in this business. However,
birds, cats and dogs in the area began to die from dehydra-
tion. Of the eighty-five horses kept there to be trained,
forty-three died within a year. It was not long before the
owners of the stables began to suffer headaches, chest pains
and severe diarrhea.

Several studies were conducted in an effort to find out
what was causing this situation. It was discovered that the
oil poured on the soil contained dioxin, a highly toxic conta-
minant that had not been removed from the oil before it was
applied to the ground.

Toxic wastes are substances generated by industry, agriculture or the government that must be disposed of in a specific
fashion as regulated by the government due to the potential
harmful effects they can have on humans. It is estimated that a
ton of toxic waste is produced per person every year by commercial industry in America,[1] but the U.S. military industry
generates about one ton of toxic waste *every minute.*[2]

In America, the incidence of environmental disease is much higher in areas near stockpiles of toxic materials.[3] Experience has shown that poor management of toxic waste is extremely expensive to correct. In spite of the efforts to control the disposal of this waste, many countries do not have sufficient infrastructure, either administrative or technological, to ensure it is done properly.

Sometimes, when the regulations for disposal become too stringent in their own country, they seek to dump waste in other countries that have no experience handling these dangerous materials: "Mexican border towns are being affected by toxic waste illegally dumped by U.S.-owned maquiladora industries."[4]

AIR POLLUTION

IN OUR WORLD today it is becoming increasingly difficult to step outside to get a "breath of fresh air." The industrialized world around us pours tons of sulfur dioxide and other toxic substances into the air each day. As we go about our lives, we don't think about the toxic gases in the air we breathe. Yet, we know that these toxins undermine the health of the populous, because every day we hear more about pulmonary diseases, allergies and fatigue.

In 1990 the government of Mexico City revealed that its steadily increasing air pollution was seriously jeopardizing the health of the city's inhabitants. One-fifth of the national population, some twenty million people, live there. It is also home to three million motor vehicles, thirty thousand industrial enterprises and twelve thousand service enterprises. Some 13,500 tons of contaminants were being produced there each day in 1990, more than in any other city in the world.[5] That is a frightful figure when you consider that the Environmental Protection Agency is very concerned because 74,000 tons are produced daily in the *whole* United States, with its hundreds of industrialized cities.[6]

Thousands of toxic elements are introduced into the air from motors, petroleum refineries, the chimneys of the chemical industry, to mention a few. This filthy soup known as smog is a product of hydrocarbon, nitrous oxide and other particles that, upon being exposed to sunlight, become toxic. Although some countries such as Japan, Germany and the United States have established standards to control toxic emissions, many other developing countries have not.

The main source of the toxic emissions that give rise to smog are motorized vehicles. A study by the University of Southern California demonstrated the damage done by smog. Researchers performed autopsies on one hundred young auto accident victims from the Los Angeles area. They found severe smog-related damage to the lungs of all these young people. The chief researcher stated that young people who live in large cities are literally having their lungs destroyed.[7]

Our bodies are not designed to expel smog particles. Thankfully, some of the toxins are eliminated by the kidneys. But the smog particles that are not eliminated often pass into the bloodstream and accumulate in fatty tissue and other cells. This causes all kinds of often irreversible damage, not only to humans, but also to animals and plants.

The illnesses traced to this pollution include difficulty breathing, vertigo, headaches, laryngitis, eye irritation, nausea, asthma, bronchitis, pulmonary emphysema, pneumonia, lung cancer, vascular diseases, skin diseases, reduction of red blood cells, lead damage to kidneys, mental retardation, sterility and high-risk pregnancies. In 1940 the visibility in Mexico City was ten miles; now it is less than two.

NUCLEAR WASTE

RADIOACTIVE PARTICLES INTRODUCED into the environment from

nuclear explosions and nuclear power plants have worried physicists for decades. Communities in the United States have complained about the number of nuclear tests performed in the deserts of Nevada and Utah since 1950. For many years, there has been evidence that it is dangerous to be exposed to the residue of such detonations.

Yet, no remedial action was undertaken by the United States government until 1984, when a federal judge in Utah ruled that ten persons had developed cancer as a result of the radiation produced by military testing. One year later, British courts held their military industry responsible for the elevated incidence of cancer in veterans who had taken part in the testing of nuclear arms at Christmas Island in 1950.

After a nuclear explosion, the atoms of uranium and plutonium produce around three hundred radioactive isotopes.[8] This radioactive conglomerate is trapped in the atmosphere and descends slowly to the ground in a radioactive rain. All creatures, especially human, are very sensitive to these radioisotopes. They invade our bodies through the air, water and contaminated foods. Even though some of them are fleeting, most will stay in the earth almost forever. For instance, the half-life of a carbon-14 isotope is 5,760 years!

On April 26, 1986, in Chernobyl, Ukraine, the world was shaken by the worst nuclear industrial accident in history. The explosion contaminated the atmosphere with 100 million curies of radioisotopes that spread from Ukraine to Great Britain.[9] Only thirty-one persons died in the explosion, but the number of deaths from the radiation introduced into the environment from the accident is impossible to calculate.

Ten thousand deer had to be sacrificed in Europe because they ate contaminated feed from the radioactive rain that will remain for at least thirty years.[10] The issue is not that the Europeans were deprived of this delicacy, but that they, along with their crops and soil, were bathed with this rain. The effects will linger for decades, because long-term exposure to small doses of radiation can cause serious illness.[11]

One of the contaminants was the well-known strontium-90, an isotope that has been widely researched because it easily contaminates milk. In cases where animals or humans are exposed to it, the incidence of leukemia and cancer of the bone is significantly higher than the rest of the population.[12]

Governments have placed a lot of emphasis on protecting the environment from nuclear contamination, and developed countries have budgeted enormous amounts for this purpose. Yet, contamination of the world's water by nuclear elements is ever increasing.

Countries that handle nuclear materials aren't careful enough disposing of radioactive waste. For instance, the Breast Cancer Incidence Study was initiated by an organization within the Department of Energy to study the higher incidence of breast cancer among female employees in the nuclear trades.[13]

Radioactive waste dumps near human settlements can be stopped if there is sufficient awareness and will to take the necessary measures. An example is the case of Sierra Blanca. Americans appealed the U.S. government to abstain from establishing a nuclear waste dump in Sierra Blanca, Texas. Mexican groups supported them since the proposed project would affect also the health of the population in the border zone. "People organized in peaceful, non-violent struggle are a powerful weapon."[14]

Indoor Pollution

To avoid smog, people stay in enclosed places. However, enclosed spaces aren't free from pollution either. When customers and employees of a bank in Encino, California, experienced headaches, nausea and vomiting, officials determined that the cause was an excessive concentration of carbon monoxide, twenty times more than the concentration accepted in smog-contaminated air![15]

In the future it is possible that indoor contamination might become a greater problem than outdoor contamination. Allergist Dr. Alfred Zamm discovered that the air inside the typical American home contains "carbon monoxide, nitric acid, and nitrogen dioxide in concentrations up to four times the maximum accepted by federal guidelines."[16]

Asbestos, highly prized for its cost effectiveness and resistance to heat, is in a lot of buildings in America, particularly schools. In the United States about fifteen million children are exposed to it, and yet, it is a proven cause of asbestosis, malignant mesothelioma and lung, mouth, larynx, esophagus, stomach, kidney and colon cancer.[17] Developed countries have started to abandon the use of this material(too late for the eleven million people who will die from cancer caused by asbestos products.

Experts calculate that we are in constant contact with some thirty-four thousand highly toxic man-made products that our body cannot metabolize or neutralize.[18] The threat is real because many of these products are found within the confines of our own homes, schools, churches, theaters, stores and offices.

THE FOODS WE EAT

YEARS AGO, WE produced food to survive; now we produce food to make money. Modern agriculture has become a lucrative industry, forever on the lookout for ways to become even more profitable.

In the food business, productivity (and profit) is increased by manipulating nature with chemical fertilizers to shorten the harvest time and with pesticides to diminish losses. Profit can also be increased by transforming perishable food into nonperishable food. But the very methods used to increase productivity and profit also severely damage or virtually erase the nutritional value of the food. These high-profit, processed foods(the backbone of the food industry(are so unnatural and unnutritional that they represent an authentic health risk.

But our bodies need real and nutritious food to meet the challenges of modern existence. Contrary to popular beliefs, eating is not just a recreational activity. Most people don't spend a great deal of time considering the nutritional quality of the foods they consume. For many individuals, this can prove to be a fatal mistake. Isn't it ironic that fast food, designed to save minutes in our day, ultimately steals years from our lives? Know your foods!

WHAT'S IN YOUR MEAT?

EXPERTS SAY THAT a creature with canine teeth is designed to eat meat. I have no desire to get into trouble with vegetarians, but people have canines. Unfortunately, we eat meat as if our canine teeth were a yard long! To supply the enormous demand, the meat industry has developed scientific methods to increase the production of red and white meats.

For decades, health authorities have told us that we need to consume all the protein we can to supply our body's needs. Meat producers responded to the challenge with flying colors (and artificial colors, too!). Dairy products have also been promoted by dieticians and nutritionists as vital. Everybody needs milk, right?

In 1940 more than four pounds of feed were needed to produce one pound of meat; in the 1980s only two pounds were necessary.[19] Fifty years ago, a cow produced two thousand pounds of milk per year. Presently, the average milk producers get fifty thousand pounds per year per cow.[20] Now, that's what I call efficiency!

The Hope of Living Cancer Free

In my opinion, meat and milk production represent one of the marvels of applied technology. Chemically enhanced feeds, genetic engineering, drugs and hormones are some of the tools used by the modern livestock industry to create the super chickens and monster cows. Dr. Frankenstein's cry "It's alive!" would have been repeated had he witnessed this frightening technology.

Consumers now have the information about what they are ingesting, thanks to recent FDA labeling regulations. But in spite of strong complaints, the livestock producers do not have to list the ingredients of their products. You may think that milk is milk, but the FDA allows the administration of up to eighty-two drugs to cows in the production of dairy products.[21] Of course, according to the industry, they are beneficial.

Antibiotics

Excessive use of antibiotics, both for prevention and treating animal infections, has become an efficient and profitable measure for the food industry—and drug companies as well. "Almost half of the 50 million pounds of U.S.-produced antibiotics is used in animals. Eighty percent is used not to treat sick animals, but instead to promote animals' growth by adding small doses into their feed."[22] Yet, the antibiotics we ingest in the foods we eat have deleterious effects, such as destruction of friendly bacteria. Because of our constant inadvertent and involuntary consumption of antibiotics in meat and milk, as well as the ones prescribed, new and resistant stains of bacteria are developing.

Nitrites

Nitrites, widely used in lunch meats, hot dogs and bacon, are another pillar of the meat industry. They not only preserve meat longer, but they also give it a cosmetic appeal by intensifying the red color. When heated, nitrites become carcinogenic. Children who eat twelve or more hot dogs a month are 9.5 times more prone to get leukemia.[23] When mothers consume hot dogs during pregnancy, the incidence of brain cancer in their offspring is greatly increased.[24]

Growth hormones

Bovine Growth Hormone and estrogen used in cattle are the most abused drugs. Their synergistic, or combined, effect provokes problems in humans such as arthritis, obesity, glucose intolerance, diabetes, heart disease and other problems less serious but annoying like headaches, fatigue, vision impairment, dizziness, menstrual problems and loss of sexual drive.

Of all the drugs used to fatten livestock and tenderize their meat, the most harmful to humans is the female hormone estrogen. When we consume commercial meats, we ingest hormones that were given to the animals in the meat production process. Excess estrogen levels in both men and women have been linked to certain types of cancer.[25]

Our world is unnaturally swarming with estrogen and estrogen-like substances. As I mentioned previously, just about all our foods contain pesticides, most of which have the chemical structure of estrogen and, when ingested, provoke a weak estrogenic effect on our systems. Other estrogen impostors come from the petrochemical industry in the form of plastics used for baby bottles and other items. Because of their weak effect, they are considered safe. But when synergism takes place, when these pesticides are combined, the negative effects to our organisms can be devastating. "Man-made chemicals used in plastics, pesticides and detergents that mimic the action of estrogen have become associated with a decline in sperm counts and an increase in breast and testicular cancers."[26]

Research overwhelmingly supports the idea that estrogen increases the incidence of many female ailments, including cancer of the breast, uterus and ovaries, among others. For instance, the extremely high incidence of breast cancer in Long Island, New York, caught the attention of National Cancer Institute researchers. They are now looking into the connection between the pesticides used on the farming soils before they were transformed into urban communities and the high incidence of breast cancer. Now the pesticides are abundant in the local tap water.

Breast tumor biopsies of women from Long Island showed unusually high concentrations of the pesticides DDT and DDE, according to Mary Wolf, M.D., a professor at Mt. Sinai School of Medicine in New York. The incidence of cancer was four times higher in these women than in women whose biopsies indicated low or no concentrations of pesticides.[27]

Western women enjoy unrestrained consumption of animal proteins and fats, along with refined carbohydrates. This diet not only increases their risk of colon cancer, it substantially increases the production of estrogens. This excessive estrogen, which is normally eliminated through the stool, is trapped in the colon because of constipation and is easily reabsorbed into the bloodstream, which already has too much.

CONTAMINATED FRUITS AND VEGETABLES

THE EASIEST WAY to transport nutrients from the soil to our bodies is by consuming fruits and vegetables. However, these fresh, perishable foods are quite vulnerable to attacks from a whole variety of natural factors(from bacteria to insects to decomposition.

These factors have always been a big concern for the food industry, which wages war with all kinds of pesticides in order to "protect" the consumer. The truth is, they are protecting their crops, but consumers pay the price by being exposed to these chemicals.

To grow the vegetables and fruits bigger and faster, indiscriminate amounts of fertilizers are dumped into the soil. As soon as the harvest is complete, the soil is prepared for the next crop. Abuse of our soil and the excessive use of fertilizers and pesticides erode it and strip it of its nutrients.

The most frequently used fertilizers destroy iron, vitamin C, folic acid, minerals, lysine and many other amino acids and nutrients. Pesticides contaminate the soil and take a long time to disappear. For example, chlorodine has a half-life of twenty years. Remember that all plants absorb the substances found in the earth. Of course, eating fruits and vegetables that contain industrial chemicals is downright dangerous

The problem is that fruits and vegetable are not just layered with pesticides on the outside. Since the pesticides go into the soil, the fruits and vegetables, which draw their minerals and nutrients from the soil, also draw in the pesticides. So these foods are internally saturated with pesticides.

While authorities have prohibited the use of some strong carcinogenic pesticides, the weak carcinogenic pesticides are still considered safe. The problem is that in laboratories, the pesticides are tested individually, but farmers normally use them in combinations because of their synergistic effects; this also increases their carcinogenic potential a thousandfold.

It's frightening to think that not only our fruits and vegetables are exposed to pesticides, but the majority (94 percent) of commercial foods are also contaminated with them.[28] Without a doubt, continuous exposure to them can cause cancer and other degenerative diseases.[29]

In 1968 a research group found that patients who died from liver cancer, brain cancer, multiple sclerosis and other degenerative diseases had significantly higher traces of pesticides in their brains and fatty tissue than did patients who had died from other types of diseases.[30]

Crushing evidence of pesticide toxicity is forcing the industry to look for new methods for protecting consumers.

This progressive industry has turned to modern-age technology and is now using radiation to sanitize produce. But radioisotopes not only destroy nutrients; they are also particles that easily enter our cells, increasing the risk of mutation and cancer.

REFINED FOOD PRODUCTS

REFINED SUGAR, REFINED flour and processed oils are the clearest examples of manufactured foods. They are the core products of the food industry. They cost almost nothing to produce, they have a long shelf-life and, because they are indispensable ingredients in all processed foods, their demand and profitability are scandalous. In fact, the crowning achievement in the food industry was the discovery two hundred years ago that it was possible to "purify" sugar of any elements that might decompose it—without taking away its sweetness. This process was called "refining."

Sugar

Since its invention in 1751, refined sugar has been the most consumed food product worldwide. However, the refining process strips the sugar cane of all its nutritional value. Refined sugar is composed of 96 percent sucrose, 3 percent waste, 1 percent water, and zero nutrients. Its calories are stripped of nutrients. Refined sugar is the prototype of foods without nutritional density. Foods with naked, or empty, calories are also known as "anti-nutrients" because, on top of not providing nutrients, they draw from stored nutrients such as thiamin, riboflavin and niacin just to be utilized!

There is a direct relationship between the explosion of chronic diseases in the 1940s and the industrialization of sugar in the 1920s. A diet that consists mainly of sugar can bring on many illnesses, including neurosis, hypoglycemia, diabetes mellitus, cancer of the biliary tract, colorectal cancer, arthritis, arteriosclerosis, coronary insufficiency and others.

Public awareness about sugar has had a positive impact, and the consumption of sugar is rapidly declining. In response to that, the food industry has increased the utilization of refined sugar in all processed foods (even salty foods) by 100 percent. Refined sugar is now ubiquitous. The average American consumes 170 pounds a year, and a whopping 82 percent comes from camouflaged sugar in processed "unfoods!"[31] Even with the improvement, sugar still constitutes 25 percent of all the calories the average person ingests.[32]

People who eat less sugar per year have a lower incidence of illness and live longer. The Seventh Day Adventists, for example, eat a vegetarian diet, and they avoid preservatives and refined foods. It is no coincidence that they live an average of twelve years longer than the rest of the population.

Refined flour

For many generations wheat has been the basis of many diets in many cultures. It is one of the main sources of protein, amino acids, complex carbohydrates and fiber. But we don't get all the benefits we used to from wheat because most of the wheat we eat now is "refined."

In the process of refining, wheat loses about 82 percent of vitamin B_1 (thiamin); 67 percent of B_2 (riboflavin); 80 percent of B_3 (niacin) and B_6; 98 percent of vitamin E; 90 percent of minerals and micronutrients; 80 percent of biotin; 76 percent of vitamin K; 75 percent of folic acid; 50 percent of linoleic acid; 85 percent of its fiber. It also loses about twenty-seven other nutrients.[33] But the virtual extraction of fiber is the greatest problem with refinement.

Our health depends on our capacity to nourish ourselves and eliminate waste. Fiber has the life-preserving task of helping our bodies eliminate waste. The result of a fiber-poor diet is a chronically constipated society.

Research groups like H. S. Goldsmith (*Lancet,* 1975) and Reddy and Wynder (*Journal of the National Health Institutes,* 1975) reported that Westerners produce small amounts of feces every twenty-four to forty-eight hours, and that their stools are hard, segmented, frequently painful and difficult to excrete. On the other hand, eaters of primitive diets eliminate three times as much waste with soft, voluminous feces that are easy to excrete.

One of the chief ways that we detoxify our bodies is thorough bowel movements, urination and sweating. If a person is constipated, that person is not excreting toxins. The longer the constipation lasts, the more toxic the person becomes. Plus, one of the chief ways to excrete estrogen is through the bowels. A constipated person is not excreting enough, so it is reabsorbed, increasing the risk of cancer. Groups of Africans, South Americans and Japanese who live in rural areas and eat primitive diets, which consist of mainly vegetables, fruits, grains rich in fiber and seldom any animal products, have almost no risk of ever developing cancer.

As you can see, we can make personal choices to help restore our bodies from the effects of environmental assaults. We can control what we eat, but some of the factors are beyond our control. I believe each of us should do our part since, no matter what, we will be exposed to external stress.

GENETICS

IT HAS BEEN estimated that about 25 percent of breast cancers diagnosed before age forty are because of mutations in a particular gene known as BRCA1.[34] After this was discovered in 1994, a similar gene, called BRCA2, was discovered.[35] Women who suffer a change (mutation) in these genes have an increased risk of breast cancer and ovarian cancer.[36]

Genetic tests are now available for detecting mutations in these genes, but since the mutations depend on several factors, it is difficult to predict who will actually get cancer. Other factors must be taken into account, such as the family history of breast cancer.

Some believe that a cancer gene can be handed down generation to generation. I believe that what is being handed down is poor eating habits as well as other lifestyle choices. A man whose mother had cancer of the colon would be likely to get it as well because they were eating at the same table for many years, right? I believe that lifestyle choices are a heavier factor than genetics.

OTHER CANCER RISK FACTORS

1. Consuming alcohol
Experts cannot explain the relationship between alcohol consumption and breast cancer, but statistics indicate that women who drink alcoholic beverages have a higher incidence of breast cancer.[37] Alcohol may also increase the production of estrogen. I have observed that alcohol can also play a role in an increase in the rate of breast cell proliferation, and it may be carcinogenic as well.

2. Smoking cigarettes
Breast and lung cancer rates started climbing at the exact same time as the sexual revolution. That's when women began doing the same stressful things that men were doing: high-stress jobs, drinking and smoking.

Don't think that smoking is responsible for lung cancer only. As the number of women smokers has increased, so have the rates of lung, breast and ovarian cancers.[38]

3. Radiation
Moderate to high doses of radiation is known to increase

the risk of breast cancer. Since a mammogram is basically an x-ray (radiation) of the breast, I do not recommend mammograms to my patients for two reasons: 1) Few radiologists are able to read mammogams correctly, therefore limiting their effectiveness. Even the man who developed this technique stated on national television that only about six radiologists in the United States could read them correctly. 2) In addition, each time the breasts are exposed to an x-ray, the risk of breast cancer increases by 2 percent.[39]

I recommend self-examination. In fact, I recommend that husbands learn how to examine their wives. A married couple is more likely to detect a lump in the breast than is a radiologist reading a mammogram.

4. Electromagnetic fields

The National Cancer Institute and the Environmental Protection Agency have commissioned studies to investigate the connection between electromagnetic fields and cancer. Scientists are trying to find out why electromagnetic fields are detrimental to our health and how to protect us from them. Until we develop a proper line of defense, I recommend refraining from using electronic devices for extended periods of time.

Be aware of all of the possible causes of cancer. With this awareness, you can start identifying things you can do to lower your own risk of cancer and the risk of your family members.

Once cancer strikes, then what strategies are available? Let's take a look at conventional strategies and their results.

7

Strategies in Conventional Medicine

I KNEW THAT I wanted to be a surgeon from the time I was a child. I attended a Christian college in America, then a medical school in Mexico. When I was accepted as a cancer surgeon at the First University of Vienna in Austria(the finest in the world—my dream came true.

The professors were patient with me as I learned German on the fly, and they placed me where language demands were minimal: the operating room. I spent more time there performing surgeries on cancer patients than any of my German-speaking classmates.

During one span of five months, I arrived at the hospital before sunup and left the operating room after sundown. I never saw sunshine during that time, and I was actually a bit traumatized by that. That is why the surgical suites at my hospital all have large windows that let "natural therapy" shine in.

I trained in conventional medicine throughout my surgical training in oncology. My father was trained as a conventional doctor as well, with a specialty in pathology. But he incorporated alternative therapies, such as megadoses of vitamins, early on. I have worked with him since 1983, and together we have become known more for alternative medicine than anything else.

We have used or tested all types of treatment methods—both orthodox and unorthodox—and we agree that there is good and bad in both worlds. I believe it is more important how and why a doctor uses a therapy than whether it is conventional or alternative.

In this chapter and the next, I will give you an overview of strategies used in the treatment of cancer, both conventional and alternative. I will share with you what treatment options are out there, but I will not counsel you on what therapy would be right for you or your loved one. A personal relationship with a competent physician is a vital part of making informed decisions about a therapy plan. Remember, doctors are similar to politicians in that each one of us has a different opinion or plan on how to resolve difficult situations.

In the last few decades the treatment of breast cancer, for instance, acquired a multidisciplinary twist. A committee consisting of a surgeon, a radiation specialist and an oncologist planned the treatment strategy to be used in "attacking" the cancer. This multidisciplinary focus continues to this day.

The first option often explored is surgery.

SURGERY

WE HAVE ALREADY discovered that much of conventional cancer therapy is based on the theory that tumors are the disease, and they should be destroyed. There are several means to achieve the removal or destruction of invasive, malignant clusters of cells from the organism. The most primitive is surgery.

Literally hundreds of procedures have been developed to remove tumors from all parts of the anatomy. Tumors may be so large and in such intricate parts of the body that through skill and experience, a surgeon must come up with an individual technique to remove a specific tumor. This is my specialty, and it is as exciting as it is challenging.

Sometimes there is little that surgery can offer. At other times, surgeries lasting twelve or more hours are needed to remove complicated tumors. But when a tumor can be removed with success, it grants the patient the best possibility of recovery. Believe it or not, surgery is the least aggressive of the orthodox treatments.

Surgery can be a helpful and compassionate cancer treatment, depending on the circumstance. If one of my patients has an obstructed intestinal track, I would not give him carrots to eat or tell him that juicing those carrots will cure him. They might even kill him. In his case, surgery would be a lifesaver.

I am alarmed, however, at how aggressive some surgeons have become. We need to be conservative about when and how we suggest a surgery. Any type of surgery is stressful on a patient and has risks.

Early cancer surgery

The idea that cancer grows by spreading its "tentacles" far and wide came from William Halsted (1852–1922), considered the father of surgery in the United States, and anthropologist Rudolph Virchow.

We can follow the history of cancer surgery by looking at cancer of the breast. In Halsted's day, breast cancer was treated either by extricating the tumor itself or by removing the entire breast. Cancer of the liver and lungs, they believed, arrived directly through these "tentacles" from the breast to the organs. Therefore, the maximum possible amount of tissue in which such "tentacles" might be hidden had to be removed.

Based on this theory, Halsted expanded the techniques he

had learned in Germany and began to practice radical mastectomy, an operation that involved the removal of the entire breast, much of the surrounding tissue, the adjacent muscles of the chest and all the lymph nodes in the armpit.

Halsted's radical mastectomy procedure was widely accepted in the United States and Europe. His approach became a teaching model for surgery in the United States. The philosophy and technique of radical surgery for breast cancer was soon applied to other kinds of malignancies as well.

Evidence for metastasis

Cancerous cells are spread to distant organs from the original tumor via the bloodstream (called "metastasis"), according to a theory published in 1910 by James Ewing of New York Memorial Hospital. Therefore, Virchow and Halsted's "tentacle" theory fell into disrepute.

Metastasis and recurrence constitute a surgeon's nightmare. Although it was proven that radical surgery wasn't necessary because there were no tentacles to remove, surgeons still blamed themselves for not removing enough tissue when tumors recurred. Many surgeons respond in the same way today. As a consequence, even more radical surgical techniques were developed. To date, these drastic surgeries are still performed without any "scientific" foundation.

Breakthroughs in conservative surgery

The disfigurement and pain of radical surgery stirred up a controversy. During the 1950s a group of surgeons questioned Halsted's ideas about radical surgery. George Crile of the Cleveland Clinic, a practitioner of radical surgery, discovered the powerful results of a British surgeon, Geoffrey Keynes, in the practice of conservative surgery. Crile convinced his colleagues to allow him to follow the conservative strategy. Crile became the first physician in the United States to attempt a clinical trial with conservative surgery for breast cancer.

The women who took part in this breakthrough strategy received partial mastectomies. Crile removed all of the tumor and an ample margin of healthy tissue. Crile's results were powerful. The gentler method proved just as successful as radical surgery. Crile exposed the medical establishment and was censored as an extremist—just an inch away from being a quack.

The breach between the defenders of radical surgeries and the defenders of the conservative type began to widen. Surgery became even more aggressive. Halsted's mastectomy expanded to include removing not only the entire breast, chest muscles and lymph nodes of the axillae, but also all the lymphatic ganglia under the sternum. This left the thorax of the patient looking like a washboard because the ribs were then only covered by the skin.

The big-shot surgeons constantly pressed for more extensive surgeries, inventing the "super-radical mastectomy." In this procedure, the clavicle was fractured and the first rib removed in order to allow doctors to cut out more tissue more easily. Fortunately, this procedure was soon abandoned due to its disastrous results, largely due to the psychological impact of the mutilation.

During the 1960s a resurgence of enthusiasm for conservative breast surgery occurred. Physicians leaned toward less aggressive surgery and the literal preservation of the breast, which meant that only the tumor was removed. This procedure was referred to as a local extrication, tumorectomy, lumpectomy or nodulectomy. When it was necessary to take away a part of the breast, it was called a partial mastectomy.

In 1964 the first major scientific study of conservative surgery for breast cancer was initiated. The study compared the removal of the tumor (local extrication) coupled with low doses of radiation therapy against radical mastectomy. The study concluded that the life expectancy of patients treated with conservative surgery and radiation was the same as those who underwent radical mastectomies.[1] This study, which was carried out in Guy's Hospital in London, was severely criticized, and the conservative movement suffered a costly setback.

It was at this point that George Crile of the Cleveland Clinic decided to take part in the debate. In 1965 Crile published a record of his experiences and continued to insist that conservative treatment was safe and effective.[2]

Evidence abounded of the fear that a conservative treatment might alter the status quo. At Harvard University, Oliver Cope, who practiced conservative surgery, wrote about his experiences to the *New England Surgical Study* (1967), but he was denied publication in their magazine. But in spite of the opposition from the proponents of radical surgery, the conservative forces gained influence and generated support from others who opposed radical surgery.

Meanwhile, in 1963 some physicians sought a balance between the two positions and suggested the removal of the breast and the armpit lymph nodes without removing the pectoral muscles. Although this made the procedure more difficult, the results were more aesthetically pleasing. This method has been referred to as a "modified" radical mastectomy. It has been well accepted internationally, but it still involves the often unnecessary mutilation of the body.

A new strategy in cancer surgery

In 1957 Dr. Bernard Fisher of the University of Pittsburgh organized a multi-institutional group called National Surgical Adjuvant Breast Project (NSABP). Fisher formed this group to study the several aspects of mammary cancer because he was not convinced of the validity of Halsted's idea that radical mastectomies were essential. Through a series of studies the NSABP successfully refuted many of the ideas of Halsted's hypothesis. No other institution or individual has contributed more to the understanding of cancer than have Dr. Fisher and the NSABP.

Findings of the NSABP

- Cancer cells do not follow an orderly pattern, but break away from the tumor and travel through the lymph nodes.

- Lymphatic lymph nodes do not impede the passage of tumor cells, but often aid the spread of the cancer. Their infection is an indication of a weak immune system.

- The condition of the patient directly influences every aspect of the tumor's progress.

- The bloodstream acts as a "highway" for cancer cells to spread throughout the body.

- Cancer cells begin to circulate at a very early stage. Cancer is a systemic disease.

- Local treatment has little effect on a patient's chances for survival.

Halstead's Hypotheses

- Tumor cells are only spread by direct extension, and they spread in an orderly manner.

- The network of lymph nodes act as barriers to the passage of tumor cells and are not involved in the spread of the disease.

- Tumors grow and spread on their own, and the

patient's condition does not influence this process in any way.

- The bloodstream does not play an important role in the spread of cancer cells.

- Tumors remain isolated and encapsulated inside the body for a long time.

- Surgical treatment is very important to the survival of the patient.

Halsted believed that it was absolutely necessary to remove the lymph nodes when treating breast cancer. In an NSABP study, surgeons treated more than a thousand women with mammary cancer, none of whom had cancer that had spread to the lymph nodes. The patients were divided into three groups: patients treated by radical mastectomy, patients treated by simple mastectomy with radiation therapy on the lymph nodes and patients treated by simple mastectomy without radiation to the lymphatic ganglia.[3]

Approximately 18 percent of the patients treated experienced cancerous spread to the lymph nodes. The surprising thing was that the survival rate was the same for all three groups. Therefore, it became apparent that there was no advantage gained when the lymph nodes were removed by surgery or treated with radiation.

The myth that lymph nodes needed to be removed, which was forwarded by proponents of radical surgery, was completely discredited. A cancer patient's prognosis does not improve with more surgical aggression. The NSABP concluded that surgeons can leave the lymph nodes alone, even when they harbor cancerous cells, without jeopardizing the patient's chances for survival.

It is true that 20 percent of the patients treated with conservative surgery experience recurrences, but it is also true that they can be treated with another conservative operation. Although 20 percent seems like a high percentage, remember that 80 percent are spared a devastating operation that would severely reduce the quality of their lives. Vera Peter, M.D., of Toronto, considered that "although the rate of recurrence is significantly higher in patients treated with conservative surgery, their life expectancy is the same."[4]

In 1985 the NSABP published the first results of a comparative study of conservative surgical treatments (simple mastectomy, lumpectomy with post-operative radiation therapy). The study concluded that patients treated with lumpectomy, the most conservative treatment, lived as long as those who received one of the other treatments.[5]

No other cancer has been as thoroughly studied as breast cancer. Yet when a patient with breast cancer is given the option for conservative surgery, like lumpectomy, she often expresses a preference for the radical approach. Why? Because surgeons often present the conservative option as "risky," claiming that there is still insufficient data to support it as the best approach.

As we close this century, radical surgery is still (incredibly) the favored approach for the treatment of breast cancer. Nevertheless, this approach is in the process of being modified, and the conservative approach is gaining acceptance.

The behavior of recurring tumors is a mystery. Some surgeons think that leaving a few cancerous cells to roam about after surgery is a deadly mistake. Others believe that these cells simply turn into tumors that can be removed without threatening the life of the patient. Still, many leaders in the field of oncological surgery, either out of fear or arrogance, continue to demand that more studies be conducted before modifying the traditional treatments.

The Hope of Living Cancer Free

CHANGING OUR THINKING ABOUT SURGERY

SIXTY YEARS AFTER the discovery that tumors spread by means of the bloodstream, we still won't change our surgical criteria. How is that possible? What justification could we possibly have to continue mutilating people when scientific, clinical studies prove that such a course of action is absolutely unnecessary?

Little has changed from the oncology of the last century and the present one, because its main instrument continues to be the scalpel. Today, when tumors are found in the early stages, surgery is considered the only effective weapon. If the patient does not end up mutilated, surgery is also considered the least aggressive treatment.

Since 1965 my father, based on the studies of Crile and others, has denounced these procedures. Like others before him, he was strongly criticized and condemned as both a "quack" and an ignoramus in oncology.

One can only hope that the medical establishment will eventually give the credit to the "quacks" who pioneered such valuable research. The promoters of a new and revolutionary idea are villainized, then ridiculed and ostracized. When change is finally embraced as valuable, the people who acted as the sharpest opponents against it often take credit for the idea.

CHANGING OUR THINKING ABOUT RADIATION THERAPY

RADIATION THERAPY IS the second line of attack. For a short time, total body radiation was used; however, that was stopped when many patients died from extreme toxicity. Now radiation therapy has evolved into a localized therapy in which dosages, as well as the size of the fields (areas where the radiation is beamed), have diminished significantly. X-ray-type beams are used to actually burn

114

malignant cells. There are adverse reactions to the therapy because, even though the fields are limited, the beam will go (within the field) through benign as well as malignant cells.

Radiation therapy, in which we placed so much faith a few decades ago, has proven to be another medical blunder. Motivated by the desperation of failure, radiation therapists have dreamed up new ways of applying increasingly aggressive doses to their patients. They have literally "burned" patients, leaving many permanently disabled. Plus, these patients have had to experience the temporary side effects of severe nausea, malaise, loss of appetite and the loss of other functions.

Radiation doses have to be specifically measured, and there is an air dose, a skin dose and a tumor dose. The calculation has to be done by an expert, many times by a physicist. The radiation therapist does the planning to prevent the burning of the skin. The lighter the skin, the more it will be affected.

According to Dr. Mario Soto, when the field of entry is large, there will be side effects. For example, if the esophagus is touched during radiation to the chest, esophagitis, or the burning of the inside of the lining of the esophagus, can result. In the case of cancer of the cervix or the uterus, proctitis, or the burning of the lining of the rectum, can be caused. In radiation to the head and neck, if radiation is given to the tongue, the salivary glands can be impacted, and the patient will be without saliva.

Each phase has to be analyzed and individualized to see if there are benefits to the patients. As the Europeans say, "Why should we cause symptoms when the patient doesn't have any symptoms?"

Changing Our Thinking About Chemotherapy

In November 1998, I had a unique opportunity to sit on a

panel with renown cancer experts at a health convention called the Health Show, held in Orlando, Florida. Dr. Bernie Siegel, a friend of mine, was the moderator.

To open the discussion, Dr. Siegel held up a copy of my magazine, the *Health Ambassador*. My managing editor was surprised and elated as Dr. Siegel read the headline on the front page: "Chemotherapy, a fate worst than death."

"You see, it is negative statements like that that are counterproductive in cancer therapy," Dr. Siegel continued. "If a person wants to choose chemotherapy and believes it will help them, they can benefit from it and do well. It does not have to be a fate worse than death."

I could see my editor shrinking down in his seat in the back of the hall. Later Dr. Siegel congratulated me on the work we are doing at Oasis of Hope, so I know that he didn't think we were completely off; he just didn't agree with our headline.

Actually, I concur with Dr. Siegel. There is a time and place for everything, including chemotherapy. I have seen chemotherapy benefit a patient, especially low-dose chemotherapy that is delivered directly to the tumor. Such is not always the case, however, and many of my patients can testify that the chemotherapy seems worse than the disease.

Chemotherapy is the field of oncology that is designed to destroy tumors through chemicals given systemically, by injection or orally, or locally, by injecting the tumors directly or through a specific artery (regional chemotherapy). The many chemotherapeutic agents are designed either to destroy the malignant cells or block specific developmental cellular processes.

Chemotherapy used against cancer is aggressive because cancer is aggressive. Since very little has worked in the fight against cancer, it is no surprise that frustration drives chemotherapists to give increasingly more aggressive treatments, both in dosage and variety of substances used.

Oncologists realize that chemotherapy is the most toxic and least effective treatment. However, since something must be done for the patient, frustration often makes chemotherapy seem like the only option. So the therapists continue to rely on this destructive treatment, which borders on the sadistic.

In most cases, chemotherapy patients feel as if they are dying. The side effects have to do with the fact that chemotherapy drugs don't just attack malignant cells; they select any cells that reproduce themselves quickly. This includes the hair follicles, which is why a patient's hair falls out. The lining of the gastro-intestinal tract also reproduces very fast, so when the chemotherapy acts there, the patient becomes nauseous and vomits. The bone marrow is also a highly proliferative tissue. Chemotherapy causes what is called bone marrow depression, which can be controlled if the oncologist or hematologist is closely involved.

Patients taking chemotherapy often feel very weak, lose their appetite and often have latent side effects of lack of taste and hypersensitivity to smells to the point that they can't stand the smell of soap or cleaning fluids.

According to clinical oncologist Dr. Mario Soto of our Oasis of Hope Hospital, certain chemotherapy drugs, such as Vincristine, are neurotoxic, that is, toxic to the nerves, and can cause severe side effects in the nervous system. Other similar drugs have the same side effects such as Taxol, which is widely used. Adramyacin can be cardiotoxic, that is, toxic to the heart, and Bleomicin can cause scar tissue in the lungs.

Many of my patients would rather die than continue with such therapy, actually preferring to take their chances with cancer rather than suffering the experience of chemotherapy.

The Hope of Living Cancer Free

The results from chemotherapy

During his ten years as a statistician, Dr. Ulrich Abel discovered that the method used for treating the most commonly occurring epithelial cancers has rarely been successful. Abel published a summary of the results of chemotherapy, *Chemotherapy for Advanced Epithelial Cancer,* in 1990.[6] In it he discusses epithelial cancer, which is a type of cancer of the lungs, breast, prostate, colon and other organs. Epithelial cancers are responsible for 80 percent of the deaths attributable to cancer in the industrialized world.

Abel affirms that there is no evidence that the vast majority of chemotherapy cancer treatments exert any kind of positive influence as far as life expectancy or quality of life. This conclusion has significant impact when we remember that Dr. Abel belongs to the establishment that prescribes such treatments.

According to Abel, the "almost dogmatic belief in the efficacy of chemotherapy is generally based on false conclusions drawn from inaccurate data." After interviews with many doctors, Abel concluded that "the personal view of many oncologists seems to be in striking contrast to communications intended for the public."[7] In other words, Abel indicated that many oncologists wouldn't take chemotherapy themselves if they had cancer.

In fact, many cancer specialists would not personally take chemotherapy. Dr. Heine H. Hansen of the Finsen Institute in Copenhagen surveyed 118 doctors, many of them cancer specialists, and was shocked to find that oncologists recommend to most patients experimental chemotherapy that experts in the field would not accept for themselves. The vast majority of doctors considered most of the treatment options with more than two to six drugs to be unacceptable options if they themselves were to take part in the clinical trials.[8]

The medical establishment insists that one of the beneficial effects of chemotherapy is that it prolongs life expectancy by five years. According to Dr. Abel, this claim is clearly false. There is only evidence that chemotherapy extends life in the case of small cell carcinoma of the lung, and that improvement consists of extending life for only three months.[9]

Here are some of the findings Dr. Abel published regarding some cancers commonly treated with chemotherapy:[10]

- *Colon and rectal cancer:* There is no evidence at all that chemotherapy prolongs the life of patients suffering these malignancies.

- *Stomach cancer:* There is no evidence of effectiveness.

- *Pancreatic cancer:* The largest study was "completely negative." The patients who experienced prolonged life were those who did not receive chemotherapy.

- *Bladder cancer:* Chemotherapy is often applied but is not effective. No prospective study has been made.

- *Breast cancer:* There is no evidence that chemotherapy raises the chances for a patient's survival. Its use is "ethically questionable."

- *Ovarian cancer:* There is no direct evidence, but it might be worthwhile to research the use of platinum.

- *Uterine and cervical cancer:* There was no improvement in the survival rate of those treated with chemotherapy.

- *Cancer of the head and neck:* There was no benefit to

receiving chemotherapy in terms of survival. There was the occasional benefit of reduction of tumor size.

In the face of these facts, you may wonder where the data is that *supports* the notion that chemotherapy is beneficial! It is true that sometimes these medications do, in effect, reduce tumor size.[11] But they have no significant impact in regard to life extension, and almost always they reduce the quality of life. As a matter of fact, the cancer sometimes comes back more aggressively than ever. Even though 99 percent of a tumor is eliminated, the resistant 1 percent is often made up of the most aggressive cells.[12]

In spite of the illuminating report on chemotherapy by Dr. Abel, there does not seem to be any tendency within the medical world to use more conservative methods. The fact is that oncologists pressure their patients to begin receiving chemotherapy immediately. George Crile affirmed in his book *Cancer and Common Sense* that "those responsible for giving information to the public have chosen to use fear as a weapon. They have created a new disease called cancer phobia, a contagious disease that spreads from mouth to ear."[13]

My brother, Dr. Ernesto Contreras, Jr., an oncologist and radiation therapist, made the following observations after twenty-five years of medical practice:

> It is really frustrating to see how little we have been able to achieve in oncology. The effectiveness of the treatment against cancer is doubtful. I have treated thousands of patients, most of them in the advanced stages of cancer, and I can't say that more than 15 percent of them had positive response to an orthodox treatment. Only another 25 percent received the benefit of a temporary remission or a real alleviation of the devastation caused by the disease. Most of the remaining 60 percent felt only a slight reduction of their pain.

I can say that only in a few patients was quality of life significantly prolonged by the aggressive treatments now available. On the other hand, I have to accept, in many cases, that the remedy was worse than the disease.

I am convinced that the real and practical value of chemotherapy and radiation therapy is very limited in specific cases. As long as we are unable to find better treatments for the vast majority of patients with cancer, it is an obligation, not just an occupation, for oncologists and physicians to dedicate their efforts toward the investigation of new and alternative treatments. Only then can we hope to find more effective, less aggressive and less toxic treatments. Only then can we hope to prolong the lives of cancer patients and maintain the quality of their lives as well.

CHANGING OUR THINKING ABOUT CANCER

THE ENORMOUS FAILURE of conventional therapies are not the result of procedures themselves, but why and how they are used. First, their application is supported on a false premise: Cancerous tumors are the disease. In reality, the tumors are but a symptom of a metabolic failure that allowed them to grow. Removing or destroying tumors without taking the necessary steps to restore the organic deficiencies that caused them accounts for most cancer recurrences and deaths.

Success is measured by what happens to the tumor and not by what happens to the patient. The second reason for failure is the criteria with which surgery, radiation and chemotherapy are offered. If the cancer is aggressive, the therapy must be aggressive. Maximum tumor mass must be removed or radiated, as much as the patient can tolerate, and chemotherapy will be given.

All of these procedures, when it is understood that the

121

disease is much more than the tumor, can be useful in limited cases to diminish tumor mass. My criteria for using them is whether I would be willing to receive it myself if I were in the same condition as my patient, and whether it is going to improve quality of life. Since in most cases the answer to both questions is no, I rarely use them.

The physical distress of conventional therapies coupled with their disappointing results have caused many patients to demand alternatives. Let me share with you some of the current breakthrough strategies that are available in alternative medicine.

8

Victory Strategies Through Alternative Medicine

My FATHER WAS invited to present case studies of patients who benefited from his metabolic therapy at a world congress on cancer in South America. It is standard protocol for the presentations made at this world congress to be published in the medical industry's top journals.

This was not the case with my father. A number of objections were raised by doctors who didn't believe that alternative methods should be condoned by including them in a scientific journal. My father was asked to present his cases before a panel of oncologists at Sloan-Kettering Memorial Hospital to determine if the science behind his methods met the standards of the journal.

I accompanied my father with excitement. I thought to myself, *It will take a miracle, but this might be the opportunity for my father's therapy approach to gain acceptance in the United States.*

We arrived at a conference room with twelve doctors whose body language told me that we were doomed. My father began to present the first case, and he put up the first x-ray and explained the tumor size and location when he received the patient. Then he put up another x-ray after the patient had undergone the Contreras' metabolic therapy.

Before he could get a word out, one oncologist stood up and told my father to stop. He stepped out of the room and reappeared promptly with a set of x-rays. The doctor said to my father, "Look at this x-ray. Here my patient has tumors. Then we treated him, and look at this next x-ray. The tumor is completely gone! Look at your patient's x-ray; the tumor has grown."

My father asked the doctor, "How is your patient doing?"

The doctor replied that the patient had died.

My father explained that his patient's second x-ray had been taken eight years after the first x-ray and that the patient was still living, working and enjoying life. The oncologist told him simply that his methods could not be considered effective because the tumors were not eradicated.

The classic definition of successful cancer treatment is when a tumor is destroyed. The general condition or how the patient is feeling is of secondary concern. If the tumor continues to be active, the treatment is considered to be a failure by oncological standards, even if the patient is feeling great.

My father and I believe that the quality of life a patient has is more important than the destruction of the tumor. What do you prefer? To live ten quality years with the tumor controlled, or to go through three months of aggressive and harmful therapies that made you sick and unable to continue any normal activity, even though the statistics indicated that your chances would not be significantly improved.

We focus on maintaining the quality of our patient's lives, and we teach them how to release their fear of cancer and focus on the joy of living. We never promise a cure or tumor destruction. Instead, we teach people to coexist with cancer. When a person is completely at peace with the fact they have cancer, the stress on their immune system is lessened, and the hope of healing or spontaneous remission increases. If the cancer never goes into remission, the patient can enjoy the life he has instead of wasting it agonizing about dying.

SEEKING ALTERNATIVES

WHAT IS ALTERNATIVE medicine? In general, alternative medicine is anything that has not been tested, approved, recommended or condoned by the Food and Drug Administration (FDA) or the American Medical Association (AMA) of the United States of America. The United States' medical system is the benchmark for the rest of the world, and anything that is approved by the FDA and the AMA is automatically inducted into the conventional medical establishment, considered orthodox and accepted and approved by every other country in the world.

The idea of naturally based therapies goes back to ancient times. Until recently, all medicine was what we now call alternative medicine. But with the advent of the pharmaceutical industry, a new chapter began. Natural therapies were replaced with synthetic ones, and governments began regulating the production and use of those. Now doctors learn to identity symptoms and look up treatment options. Then they prescribe what the pharmaceutical companies and the studies say works.

Since most alternative medicines are natural, it would be unrealistic to get them approved by the FDA. Why? Well, even if it could be proven that a fruit, for instance, could cure a disease, why would anyone spend the millions necessary to get it through the FDA? There would be no way to recoup that investment because fruit is already available to everyone. So many alternative medicines remain unapproved.

It is interesting that chemotherapy is FDA approved, and yet, as we will see, reports indicate that it is toxic (harmful) and not very effective. But chemotherapy drugs are manufactured by pharmaceutical companies with the money necessary to complete all of the required tests. The objective results of tumor destruction were demonstrated adequately. But the ultimate test—whether the patient lives or not—is not one of the factors considered in clinical trials.

However, when conventional therapies failed to live up to their promise, people became extremely interested in alternative therapies. In 1994 the magazine *MPLS St. Paul* dedicated its cover to acupuncture, herbalism, therapeutic massage, macrobiotic diet, chiropractic and other therapies. In an article titled "New Ways of Healing," it was reported that even orthodox hospitals were allowing the admission of alternative services, not because they believed in them, but to regain lost clientele.[1]

The April 6, 1992 issue of *Time* magazine broke all sales records. The cover displayed a variety of vitamin tablets and capsules and bore the title "The Power of Vitamins. New research shows they may help in the war against cancer, cardiac disease and the ravages of aging."

In the face of the atrocious results of orthodox cancer treatments, the public has decided to look to alternatives criticized by the medical establishment. People are moving toward answers that are rejected by those who do research in laboratories. United States government authorities and scientists, in spite of the overwhelming quantity of studies from the world's universities, seem to want to keep us tied to the belief that nothing apart from the approved treatments is effective, and that the proposed alternative therapies lack scientific basis.

If the authorities were impartial, they would prohibit the approved treatments for cancer since, scientifically, they have been demonstrated to be useless. Beyond that, clinical studies have demonstrated that these treatments actually endanger the quality of life and are often fatal.

CONVENTIONAL AND ALTERNATIVE MEDICINE

MANY MEDICAL AUTHORITIES censure alternative therapies for several reasons. Let me address each of these objections to alternative therapy:

They promise miraculous healing and offer false hope. I agree that if someone says a particular therapy is able to cure every disease, that person has a God complex and is dangerous. Yet, supporters of orthodox medicine commit a greater wrong when they prohibit alternatives for problems for which they have nothing to offer. They assert that if orthodox medicine has not found a solution, then no one can.

A false hope is one that has neither scientific basis nor proven results. My question is, Do their scientifically proven treatments offer a true hope? Usually not. "Go home and settle your affairs, because you are going to die in a few months. Don't waste money on alternative therapies," they say. So much for hope.

They involve secret procedures or ingredients. The criticism of secrecy seems very strange to me since the foundation of modern medicine is cemented with patents that protect the secrecy of drugs. But when a medical "quack" discovers a method that promises longevity, it is judged as secretive. I will admit, however, that I believe creative methodology that helps the sick should be shared.

They involve exorbitant cost. On the issue of cost, alternative therapies are enormously cheaper than conventional ones. The cost of orthodox oncological treatments is truly exorbitant.

More importantly, most of those who consult the so-called "quacks" say they are satisfied with the treatment received. Who has to be satisfied, the authorities or the patients?

They report exaggerated positive results backed only by anecdotal case histories. Compared to orthodox therapies for chronic degenerative diseases, the results of alternative therapies are amazingly superior. Alternative therapies are backed by a multitude of studies, but these studies are often disregarded by orthodoxy.

They invite us to abandon or delay proven medical treatment. Time and time again it has been confirmed that the "proven medical treatments" are not only ineffective but also dangerous. The vast majority of patients with cancer live longer and better without the orthodox treatments.

As I have already mentioned, studies show that many oncologists would not accept their own treatments themselves. No scientific research is needed to prove that fresh vegetables, fruit, juices, medicinal herbs, vitamins, minerals and fiber are not harmful to the body. It would be nice if proof existed that surgery, radiation and chemotherapy were not harmful.

The medical establishment may criticize alternative doctors and treatments, but the fact is that more and more doctors are becoming interested in alternative therapies. Associations like the American College of Advancement in Medicine (ACAM) and other associations are jumping on the bandwagon. Hundreds of doctors are recommending or using alternative therapies in their offices, and almost all of them, according to Dr. Allan Bruckheim from Tribune Media Services, are satisfied with the results and plan to continue prescribing them.

AVAILABILITY OF ALTERNATIVE THERAPIES

ARE ALTERNATIVE MEDICINE therapies for cancer available in the United States? Yes. Some acupuncture and chiropractic procedures are cancer therapies, but they are not approved as such by the FDA. A cancer patient can undergo these therapies as long as the doctor does not specifically prescribe them as a treatment for cancer.

Many medical treatments, such as vitamin therapies and even laser surgery techniques, are being widely used in Canada, Europe, Asia, South America and Africa, but they are not available in the United States because they have not gained FDA approval.

Many Americans have awakened to this fact, and they don't like the idea that Europeans, Mexicans and people from other countries have access to medical treatments they don't. In response to that, President Ronald Reagan passed a bill giving Americans the right to seek medical care outside of United States, then return home to America with a three-month supply of that "alternative medicine," even if it is not FDA approved. Although Americans seeking alternative health care appreciate that, most people don't want to have to leave home to have access to these alternatives.

BREAKTHROUGH ALTERNATIVE STRATEGIES— WHICH TO CONSIDER

SINCE MY FATHER became so well known for alternative methods, hundreds of doctors and scientists have approached us over the years from many different countries telling us of their new miracle therapies. I must tell you that I have found a few effective therapies and a bunch that aren't worth the packages they arrive in. I will share with you my comments on a few of the most famous alternative therapies that I have either used or have seen being used in other alternative clinics, along with my impression of each.

Laetrile therapy
My father is the most famous pioneer of the use of Laetrile, also referred to as amygdalin and B_{17}. He is a hero of the healed, but he has been criticized by doctors who don't believe that Laetrile has any therapeutic value. This natural, antitumor agent has been the source of many disagreements,

but I have witnessed positive results with its use.

Chemically speaking, Laetrile is a diglucoside (a sugar) with a cyanide radical. It exists in all seeds, except citrus, and in many plants. Egyptian doctors used it for curative purposes from the time of the Pharaohs, and records show that Chinese herbalists used it in the year 2800 B.C. It is a successful but maligned alternative cancer treatment.

Researchers began studying the substance because the Hunza tribes in the Himalayas enjoy one of the lowest incidence of cancer in the world.[2] Their main source of protein is apricot kernels—one of the best sources of amygdalin.

The Pueblo Indians of Taos, New Mexico, traditionally eat many foods rich in amygdalin. Not coincidentally, cancer is also rare among this population. Robert G. Houston, who has written several articles on the Pueblos, was given a recipe by them as he researched a book on cancer prevention: In a glass of milk or juice, mix a tablespoon of honey with a quarter ounce (two dozen) freshly ground apricot kernels, or one kernel for every ten pounds of body weight. Houston wrote that the drink was so delicious he had it daily.[3]

Biochemist Dr. Ernest T. Krebs, Jr., discovered that it was amygdalin that was protecting these people from developing cancer. Krebs called it vitamin B_{17}. Later, his research group found that amygdalin has powerful cancer-killing capabilities because it contains cyanide, which destroys cancer cells.

Already judged as therapeutically ineffective, health officials claimed that Laetrile was also a poison![4] Interestingly, virtually every fruit, with the exception of citrus, contains some amount of Laetrile. To date, we have treated over forty thousand patients with high dosages of amygdalin and have never had one case of cyanide poisoning.

Krebs found enzymes that activate (beta-glucosidase) and neutralize (rhodenase) cyanide in our bodies. Cancer cells have a 3600-fold concentration of beta-glucosidase and are extremely deficient in rhodenase. That is why naturally occurring cyanide is so devastating for malignant tumors. Rhodenase, the cyanide-neutralizing enzyme, is very abundant in our bodies and detoxifies the cyanide released by foods and Laetrile. It's God's way.

"The cures for all man's diseases already exist in the world around us. It is the task of science to recognize them," said Selman Abraham Waksman, a famous pharmacology expert.[5] Amygdalin is natural chemotherapy, effective and completely nontoxic. Furthermore, when the amygdalin breaks down, it produces a very strong painkiller, another blessing for patients with tumors.

Amygdalin is extraordinarily effective in common tumors such as carcinomas of the prostate, breast, colon and lungs, as well as lymphomas. Twenty years ago, German scientists reported that enzymes that break up proteins could aid amygdalin by synergism, or by the energy released by combining them.[6] Since that time, both have been given together, resulting in an improvement of our statistics.

Let me share with you the story of one of my father's patients. My father has records of thousands of patients with similar results. This man had a primary tumor in the kidney with metastasis in the lung. He came to my father in 1987 to take Laetrile and the metabolic therapy.

If I showed you the x-rays from 1987, and from follow-up in 1994 and 1999, you could see the tumors in all of them. The patient still has tumors, but he has survived with a cancer for twelve years that should have killed him in less than twelve months. He was feeling great and going strong the last time I talked with him. In fact, he was going to give a lecture at a cancer conference.

My objective as a cancer specialist is not necessarily to get rid of cancer, but to assure that my patients have a good quality of life, however long that might be.

The Hope of Living Cancer Free

Oxygen therapy

Cancer cells do not survive well when exposed to oxygen. The world has the German physiologist Otto Warburg, M.D., to thank for this discovery. Just the opposite is true with normal cells, which thrive on oxygen. Dr. Warburg also demonstrated that healthy cells deprived of oxygen can become cancerous.[7]

Many therapies have been developed with the intent of destroying malignant cells through oxygen exposure based on Warburg's theory. Doctors have tried having patients breathe pure oxygen and have even put patients in hyperbaric chambers so they can be in a pure oxygen environment under pressure. Gas laws dictate that cells will absorb more oxygen under pressure.

Ozone is another oxygen therapy. The oxygen in the air we breathe is made up of two oxygen atoms, thus we call it O_2. Ozone is an oxygen molecule made up of three atoms of oxygen, O_3. I have seen ozone benefit patients with cancers, such as rectal and cervical, that could be accessed directly with ozone.

The greatest problem presented to developers of oxygen therapies is that no one has been able to discover how to get oxygen to the malignant cells. There seems to be a barrier that protects the cancerous cells from being penetrated by oxygen.

In January 1999, I had experience with a therapy called Kem O_2, which appears to be breaking the barrier in some cases. Kem O_2 is a liquid mineral preparation that theoretically causes malignant cells to generate oxygen within themselves, resulting in their own destruction. There are not enough documented cases to support any claims at this time, and we do not know what types of cancer might respond well to this therapy. But let me share with you a few stories of patients who have received Kem O_2 and experienced drastic improvement.

The first one is that of a seventeen-year-old boy who was diagnosed with a glyoblastoma multiforma grade four, one of the fastest-growing cancer tumors. The boy received Kem O_2, and within two months, the tumor reduced in size by more than 50 percent.

A forty-seven-year-old woman who had cancer of the breast with metastasis to the brain began taking Kem O_2 in April 1999. Just a few days later, on May 3, 1999, the x-ray showed that the tumor had almost disappeared. This was an amazing case.

Another patient had a primary tumor of the liver. It was a small tumor, but primary tumors of the liver are rare and very aggressive, and they normally grow very quickly. Just after a few days of Kem O_2, the tumor was completely gone.

The early results in 1999 are promising, but further studies must be conducted to come to any determination of efficacy.

Energy and resonance therapy

Our cells are made up of atoms that have electrons moving around rapidly. In fact, we are electrical beings, and each cell resonates (moves back and forth) at its own rate. The rate at which it moves is called its "frequency." In theory, if the frequency of a malignant cell is identified, we should be able to identify a frequency that could disrupt the resonance of that particular cell, resulting in its destruction.

The most famous scientist who worked in this field was the American Royal Rife. There are reports (or fabulous legends) that Royal Rife cured many cancer patients with his electromagnetic machine, but he passed away decades ago, and no one has an original Rife machine to my knowledge. I have tried many different machines produced by people claiming to have the original design, but none of the results have been impressive.

I have also seen other machines that use sound, light and radio waves to create frequencies. To date, I have found none of these to work. However, I believe that the greatest advances in medicine will come from this field of electromagnetic medicine. Just wait and see.

Food therapies

Some of the most famous and effective food-based therapies include the Gerson Therapy, the Hallelujah Diet and macrobiotics. I believe in and promote the concept upon which all these therapies are based. These therapies assert that the body contains toxins that bog down the immune system and make it susceptible to disease. In addition to the toxins, the immune system lacks nutrients to fight off the disease. These therapies use foods and juices to detoxify the body and load it up with nutrients.

These are vegetarian regimes, but each of them is a bit different. Meat and dairy products are strictly prohibited. Following these diets requires commitment and discipline on the part of the patient, but I have seen great benefit from them. I am saddened by patients who choose chemotherapy because it is easier than getting up and juicing fruits or vegetables a few times a day.

Charlotte Gerson (Gerson Therapy) and George Malkmus (Hallelujah Acres) are friends of mine. Perhaps they should develop a remote control to help the couch potato prepare the food and juices so more people would get started on their diets.

714X

This therapy is designed to stimulate—actually liberate—the immune system through direct injections into the lymphatic system of nitrogen-rich camphor and organic salts. We performed a small clinical trial of this therapy with a few patients and saw no benefit of 714X. But I have talked to many patients who tell me I should try it again, because others have benefited from it.

Do you remember the news story about the teenage boy from Massachusetts who had cancer and ran away from home in 1994 when the doctors wanted him to take more chemotherapy? The news agencies dubbed him, "The boy who ran away from chemotherapy." His name is Billy Best, and he is now cancer free. I met him, and he told me how he went to Canada for 714X, and it worked for him. He came to stay at my hospital for a couple of months to see how we do things. While he was here, we did lab work confirming his healthy condition.

Billy also told me that Essiac tea has been a great benefit. I am not sure about that either. Many of my patients drink it and feel great, so I cannot say that it is a waste of time.

Body/mind medicine

Therapies such as meditation, chanting, praying, laying on of hands and relaxation are all proving to have beneficial aspects to them. One of the most famous body/mind doctors is Deepak Chopra. He shares with his patients and readers Eastern philosophies, which most Christians are leery of.

Harvard University has a highly respected doctor named Herbert Benson who is heading up the investigation about the therapeutic benefits of psychological and emotional therapies for the body. He, along with Dr. Koenig from Duke University, are proving through clinical trials that people who pray or have religious beliefs recuperate faster and better from major illnesses.[8]

The problem that I have with most of the philosophies promoted by many of these doctors is that they are helping people get in touch with themselves, not Jesus Christ. I believe that all healing comes from God. Regardless of how much I get in touch with myself, if God doesn't choose to heal me, I won't get well.

So why do people benefit from prayer and relaxation if they are not focusing on Christ? In my opinion, when a person prays, relaxes or meditates, he or she benefits because these techniques help to relieve stress. Stress is so detrimental to our immune system.

My father was pioneering body/soul/spirit medicine before some of the New Age gurus of today were born. He sings, prays and tells jokes with his patients, and he shares Jesus with all of them. He lets people know that Jesus has the resources necessary to resolve their problem. So many of our patients leave their burdens at the altar.

Prayer therapy

We pray with the patients at my hospital, not as a pastime, but as a therapy. My nephew, Dr. Daniel E. Kennedy, had the vision to share this aspect of our treatment program with the world and founded the Worldwide Cancer Prayer Day on June 5, 1998. Recently he had the opportunity to write an article on prayer therapy for the Christian health magazine *Body and Spirit.* An excerpt from "Does Prayer Work?" follows:

> Prayer is regarded as the desperate act of the defeated, a last resort. Yet, if more doctors faced the facts about prayer as a healing agent, they would embrace it as a frontline defense.
>
> The research supporting the therapeutic benefit of prayer has been around for a long time. If doctors need to be convinced that prayer has medicinal value, they can consult their industry's journals. The scientific data derived from hundreds of clinical trials performed in reputable universities and hospitals have already been published.

In July of 1988, the *Southern Medical Journal* published Dr. Randolph C. Byrd's study, "Positive Therapeutic Effects of Intercessory Prayer in a Coronary Care Unit Population." Perhaps no other clinical trial on prayer has been surrounded by so much attention.

Dr. Byrd, a resident cardiologist, took 393 patients from the San Francisco General Hospital Coronary Care Unit and input their names on a computer. Then, the computer randomly divided the patients into two groups. One group, the "prayer group," was prayed for by a home group of Christians. The patients in the "control group" did not receive prayer. This double-blind study—called that because neither patient nor physician is aware of the trial—adhered to the same stringent guidelines that all pharmaceuticals undergo to evaluate efficacy.

The results showed that prayer was a significant therapeutic agent. Not one patient from the prayer group required an artificial airway and ventilator, whereas twelve from the control group did. In addition, prayer group patients were five times less likely to require antibiotics and three times less likely to develop complications than their control group counterparts. Dr. Byrd's study raised some eyebrows within the medical community.

Similar studies have been conducted since Dr. Byrd's study renewed interest in the subject. The most recent of these was conducted at Duke University by cardiologist Mitch Krucoff, M.D. He launched a pilot study of 150 angioplasty patients. The preliminary results suggested that patients who received prayer in addition to conventional medical treatment experienced a recovery that was 50 percent to 100 percent better than those patients who did not.[9]

In September 1977, the prestigious *New England Journal of Medicine* published a study comparing two groups of patients who had been recommended for bypass surgery. One group chose to forego the surgery and pray instead. The two year survival rate of the patients who underwent the surgery was 86 percent. The twoyear survival rate of the patients who chose prayer over the surgery was an astounding 87 percent.

While pharmaceutical companies have full-time sales reps and five-inch-thick books to keep physicians apprised of the prescription drugs at their disposal, is there anyone telling doctors about the therapeutic value of prayer? The answer used to be no—but times are changing. Many medical schools have added to their curriculum the study of prayer and other topics which examine the relationship between body, mind and spirit. This trend of investigation is partly due to public demand. Only 5 percent of doctors now say they should pray with their patients. But national surveys consistently show nearly 80 percent of patients want their physician to consider their spiritual needs.[10]

Prayer has therapeutic value. Scientists and skeptics may continue to explain it away if they are unwilling to embrace the existence of the loving Creator. However, for those who believe in the Almighty, there is a great deal of healing potential in prayer.

I am not a huge fan of the idea that there is a specific formula to use that will coerce God into action. But I do know that Scripture does specify what we are to do when someone is sick:

> Is any one of you sick? He should call the elders of the church to pray over him and anoint him with oil in the name of the Lord. And the prayer offered in faith will make the sick person well; the Lord will raise him up. If he has sinned, he

will be forgiven. Therefore confess your sins to
each other and pray for each other so that you
may be healed. The prayer of a righteous man is
powerful and effective.
　　　　　　　　　　　　　　　—JAMES 5:14–16, NIV

Prayer represents a powerful therapeutic force. The
Bible says so and science is busy confirming that truth.
God has always been the healing power that works
through prayer. Personally, I have witnessed spontaneous remissions as well as slow, steady improvement
as a result of prayer. I have also seen how prayer can
bring a person into a peaceful preparation for the next
life. I not only condone the use of prayer in the hospital
I work at, I am thrilled to prescribe it to all of our
patients. Prayer is effective, nontoxic and free. I know
of no other therapy that has so many positive aspects
and is totally free of negative side effects.

OTHER ALTERNATIVE THERAPIES

HERE IS A quick list of other alternative therapies to give you
an idea of how vast the field is:

Aromatherapy	Biological dentistry	Live cell therapy
Cancer vaccines	UV blood irradiation	Enzyme therapy
Fasting	Homeopathy	Hydro colonic therapy
Hyperthermia	Meditation	Visualization
Pyschoneuroimmunology		Hoxsey therapy

There are literally thousands of alternative therapies out
there, and if I were to list them all, this book would look like
a telephone book. In fact, such a book exists. It was presented by Burton Goldberg, and more than four hundred
doctors contributed to it. It contains over one thousand

pages, and it is available through his website at www.alternativemedicine.com. The book is called *Alternative Medicine, The Definitive Guide.*

Changing Attitudes Toward Alternative Medicine

I HAVE ALSO discovered that many individuals are put off by alternative medicine because they believe it is tied to the New Age movement. Let me tell you, the alternative medicine health conventions I attend are full of New Agers. Sometimes I feel like the only Christian there. They don't have a problem with me. Their general attitude is, "Oh, you are a Christian—great! You worship Jesus. I worship Buddha, a plant, Mohammed, Hari Krishna or whatever. It doesn't matter. We embrace everything—whatever makes you feel good."

Often these people are extremely healthy, and they take better care of themselves. They read the Bible, take all of the health tips, apply them and benefit from them.

Christians read the Bible and focus in on things like, "It is not what goes into our mouth that is unclean, it is what comes out of it." That way we justify eating junk food. Besides, we are going to heaven sooner or later, so why take care of our bodies?

Is working out in the gym a lot considered body worship, or idolatry? The truth is that God instructs us to take care of our bodies, the temples of God, and to keep them pure. The Bible is full of natural remedies, instructions on diet and healing techniques. Let's take advantage of the gift of wisdom and knowledge God has presented to us in the Bible.

The Best Option

IT IS NOT my objective to sway you toward alternative medicine. In fact, I oppose the labels *alternative* or *conventional* medicine.

The type of therapy we use is not as important as how we use it.

As you know, I am a conventionally trained cancer surgeon. I know that there are situations in which surgery, chemotherapy and radiation can be beneficial. But I also understand the limitations and negative side effects of these strategies. Sometimes I have used chemotherapy with my patients, specifically with patients who have metastasis to the liver. But I don't give general systemic chemotherapy. I give it in small doses directly to the tumor in the liver through a catheter that I install surgically.

One of my most famous patients was Donald Factor, the son of Max Factor. He was diagnosed with cancer in 1986. He was so sick when he arrived that I didn't know if he had a chance of surviving. We did localized chemotherapy to the tumor in his liver. He is doing extremely well now, and he is cancer free! You can read his testimony in Appendix C.

I have been greatly criticized by conventional doctors for using alternative techniques such as the one I used with Donald Factor, but then alternative doctors criticize me for using chemotherapy and surgery—even in small amounts.

Nevertheless, my deepest desire is that doctors will open their eyes to all of the possibilities and inform their patients of the option that holds the greatest promise of a quality life.

Now, let me show you how we treat cancer patients in our Oasis of Hope Hospital.

9

An Oasis of Hope

ONE MORNING A fourteen-year-old apprentice decided (while the carpenter was away) to cut a small sheet of half-inch plywood. He had seen this done many times, and he thought it looked quite easy. It took only milliseconds for the electric saw, rotating at thousands of revolutions per minute, to rip through this young man's hand. He felt only heat before his reflexes took over, and he quickly yanked his hand from the revolving teeth.

He was rushed into the operating room with an ugly cut. The wound was deep, and the index finger, hanging under the hand, was pale and quickly turning blue. I examined him under a surgical microscope to assess the possibility of saving the fingers and their function. Very often, cuts are perpendicular to the finger. Injuries like that require a clean-cut incision with relatively easy reconstruction procedures. But in this boy's case, the cut was tangential and oblique; it had consumed rather than just cut through some of the tissue. This is a great problem on the skin, but the capsule of the joint that holds the finger to the hand was almost half gone, and a good part of the bone on both ends of the joint was missing, too.

Through a miracle from God, the electric saw that had ripped through his index and middle fingers had not detached either of them. However, about one-quarter inch of the sheath that covers the tendon that moves the index finger was destroyed (an enormous breech in this part of the anatomy), and the main artery and nerve were severed. The middle finger was also in bad shape, but the artery and nerve were not severed. The tendon and bone would need some work, though.

Although I openly criticize our reliance on technology for improving the quality and length of our lives, there is no question that technological advances have brought many medical benefits to those who are privileged to have access to them.

Plastic, vascular and microsurgery were subspecialties that I thoroughly enjoyed during my training in Vienna. They are very important in cancer surgery, because sometimes large tumors in the face, neck, breast, hands or feet have to be removed, and the reconstruction has to be functional and aesthetic.

With the help of a powerful microscope, I was able to locate the severed anatomical parts and decide on a plan of action. After controlling the bleeding, I began to reconstruct the joint's capsule first, then the tendon, artery and nerve. Instruments precise enough to handle needles and threads smaller in diameter than the thinnest of hairs allowed me to mend and reconstruct this terrible wound.

Little by little I was able to get the index finger back to its original location. A healthy pink color began to appear as soon as the artery was put back together. As I attached one end of the nerve to its mate I prayed that this young man would recover some function.

The middle finger was much less work. Even though the skin tear was awful, the cut on the tendon was cleaner, and the reconstruction went smoothly.

The moment of truth arrived the next morning when the bulky bandages were removed. Both fingers looked good. The flap on the middle finger looked iffy, but there was no doubt in my mind that the fingers were going to hold.

With much reservation I asked Eduardo, the injured boy, to try to move his fingers. After painstaking effort, he was able to move them minimally. He may never be a concert pianist, but he will have a fully functional hand.

If this accident had happened in a place where no microscope and precision instruments were available, the only option would have been amputation. Thank God for technology!

Many lives are saved daily, and even more disabilities are avoided through these surgical advances. I feel blessed to be alive at this time of history.

Yet my goal continues to be helping people understand that there is no saving technology, no perfect formula, no silver bullet. Preventing cancer or putting it into remission is a complex process, and in all my years of experience and networking with other cancer specialists, I have not found one program that cures every patient.

INDIVIDUAL TREATMENT CHOICE

THERE ARE SO many variables when it comes to treating patients. You can't treat every cancer patient the same way even if they have the same diagnosis. People have different genetic traits. They come from different living environments, and they have different eating habits. Their social activities and family relationships differ; they may or may not believe in God, and they may or may not have had a recent tragedy in their lives. With all the variables, it is impossible to say that there is one cure to cancer, be it conventional, alternative, experimental, integral, complementary or holistic.

The Hope of Living Cancer Free

Cancer patients are faced with the burden of choice. The inability of medical science to provide effective therapies has opened the door to numerous options that range from the familiar to the exotic. Opposing theories and confusing treatment options add to the difficult choices. Plus, doctors and other health professionals often find it tough to come to a consensus. Even after so many decades of research and reports, oncologists from the same research institution still cannot agree on what the treatment for a specific cancer should be. This only reinforces the fact that the vast knowledge we have acquired through cancer research has brought no relief for patients or doctors.

What is the patient to do? How can we, the medical community, be more precise and effective? I don't have an easy answer. Nevertheless, let me give you some guidelines.

By now, you have information on a number of the treatment options, both conventional and alternative. The information is of value only if it is practical for you. What we have learned from years of providing alternative and complementary medicine to more than one hundred thousand patients is that no two people are alike. Each and every patient has specific needs, be they metabolic, emotional or spiritual. At Oasis of Hope we tailor the treatment according to each patient's specific needs.

Remember that cancer is triggered by exposure to carcinogens and the inability of the immune system to protect the body from the insult of the environment. Never lose sight of the fact that God established healing pathways in our organisms. Our goal is to remove obstacles, and then aid those pathways to achieve results that the patients can enjoy. Meanwhile, some treatments must be endured.

Cancer can strike at hundreds of different sites in the body. The four most common sites of cancer are lung, breast, prostate and colon. Let me share with you how we treat patients with these cancers at Oasis of Hope and what we do when cancer spreads from any of these organs to the liver (liver metastasis). These malignancies pose the greatest risk to society.

OUR GENERAL TREATMENT PHILOSOPHY

INVOLVING THE PATIENT in the decision-making process is our treatment philosophy. We never use therapies that destroy the patient's quality of life. Instead, we provide them with treatments that improve the quality of their lives.

We use orthodox treatments when absolutely necessary if they will improve the patient's health. Surgery is sometimes necessary to remove a tumor that is blocking, say, the digestive tract. In the same way, chemotherapy and radiation therapy may be helpful in specific cases. The resultant tumor reduction may not be permanent, but it gives us the time needed for the alternative therapy to work.

Patients need a treatment that will attack the root of the problem. Natural therapies destroy tumors slowly through internal mechanisms (immunities). These nontoxic therapies give the body the weapons it needs to fight illness. They do not just attack the symptoms; they truly attack the foundation of illness.

Many clinics and hospitals have "anti-tumor" programs that are inflexible. Like a shoe store that only offers one size, these programs force the patient to fit into the program. Our oncologists' mission is to find an adequate treatment specific to the needs of each patient. So, we are eclectic in our approach.

For the past thirty-six years, we've had the opportunity to evaluate many products and alternative remedies, such as shark cartilage, cat's claw, herbs, homeopathic products, nontoxic medicines, electromagnetic fields and more. We research all avenues that appear promising, have sufficient scientific basis, suggest efficacy and are nontoxic. But everything must fit into our philosophy: *The treatment must not negatively affect the quality of the patient's life, and we must use treatments we would choose for ourselves if the need arose.*

The medical industry, with its seemingly limitless treatment options, suddenly has very little to offer that meets those simple requirements. But God has provided everything we need for the maintenance of our health in nature. The most natural and least aggressive modalities are the ones we offer. We improve the patient's ability to fight disease by providing the body, mind and soul with the tools they need. In other words, we are not in the business of getting rid of tumors (and thereby, patients). God gave our bodies the capacity to heal themselves, and our mission is to provide the necessary resources for our patients to get well.

METABOLIC THERAPY—THE CONTRERAS' FOUNDATION OF HEALING

ORIGINALLY, MY FATHER called our method of treatment "holistic therapy" because he recognized that, to obtain the best results, one had to treat the patient in the physical, emotional and spiritual spheres. The term holistic has now been adopted by many followers with humanistic or anti-Christian religious philosophies. To avoid confusion, my father coined the term *metabolic therapy.*

Metabolism is the total function of the body. In order for this total function to be carried out efficiently, body, mind and spirit should work in harmony. Caring for our patients in *totality* is the goal of the metabolic therapy. This goal is achieved through several branches: detoxification, diet, immune stimulation and antitumor agents. Each has the objective of providing resources to create the best healing environment in our organism to fight off cancer, while at the same time making the cancer cells unwelcome. Let's explore these.

<u>GETTING IN SHAPE FOR BATTLE</u>

Detoxification

Our health and therefore our lives depend basically on two things: the intake of the necessary nutrients and the elimination of waste. The fact that there are more organs designated for the elimination of waste should indicate the importance of detoxification.

Many of the toxins found in the air, ground, water, food and medicines remain in our bodies, causing serious damage. At times, these poisons permanently embed themselves in our tissues. Our bodies are often so besieged by toxins that the organs designed for elimination of waste (colon, liver, kidneys, lungs and skin) are overwhelmed and incapacitated. Therefore, an integral part of metabolic therapy is detoxification.

We have developed methods that can effectively help the body get rid of these toxins. High-fiber preparations increase intestinal passage. Colonics and coffee enemas help clean the lower intestinal tract. Intravenous solutions with amino acids (EDTA) pick up toxic substances and eliminate them in the urine.

Breathing exercises and oxygen therapy are also essential parts of the detoxification process. Finally, natural substances like milk thistle and garlic increase liver detoxification.

When all these therapies are used in conjunction, the body is assisted in the task of eliminating harmful toxins that block its normal function. A "clean" body is in better shape for battle.

The Hope of Living Cancer Free

Diet

We cannot avoid the ravages of the environment, but in great measure, we can control the food we put in our mouths. While in the hospital, our patients consume natural, organically grown foods without preservatives or toxins. Whole-grain cereals, whole-grain breads and foods loaded with nutrients like vitamins, phytochemicals, flavonoids, minerals, proteins and fiber are all part of the therapy.

Malignant cells obtain their energy mainly from proteins and fats, while normal cells produce their energy almost exclusively from carbohydrates. Dr. Otto Warburg received the Nobel Prize for medicine in the 1920s for making this discovery. Few medical practitioners make use of this vital information. But based on these scientific facts, my father initiated the use of food as an anticancer therapy more than thirty years ago, recommending that his patients ingest a diet rich in complex carbohydrates (fruits and vegetables), poor in protein and very low in fat (fatty meats and milk products). God's plan is that we eat things that provide enough nutrients to prevent disease and to maintain health.

Immune stimulation

A strong immune system is vital for overcoming disease. Cancer exploits the body's weakness and inability to defend itself. In reality all diseases are opportunistic. Too often the immune systems are forced to work overtime against an environment filled with destructive and carcinogenic agents.

Even though we serve organic food to our patients, we also provide extra support through nutritional supplements. Megadoses of vitamins, minerals, phytochemicals and amino acids are administered to our patients continuously.

Since stress severely depresses the immune system, stress-reducing techniques are very important. Therefore, as part of the immune stimulation program, we offer patients psychological and spiritual counseling. All patients have the option of participating in spiritual programs where they have the opportunity to have a personal encounter with God.

With an immune-stimulated patient, the weapons aimed directly at the tumor are much more effective.

GOING TO BATTLE

CANCER HAS NO word of honor. We must use all resources at hand to combat this incredibly stubborn and effective enemy.

Remember that our goal is not to destroy tumors, but to protect a good quality of life. Nature does provide, however, a large arsenal of weapons to destroy tumors, or at least to neutralize their growth. Natural cancer-busters like Laetrile, Kem O_2, shark cartilage, garlic, vitamin A, urea and selenium are employed in the treatment course for most of our patients. We also make available whatever other therapies will improve the quality of life for our patients (low-dose chemotherapy, radiation and surgery) when a real benefit can occur.

Now that you have had an overview of our therapies that are common for most patients, let me share some of our specific treatments for various types of cancer.

SPECIFIC CANCER THERAPIES

Cancer of the lung

Lung cancer is the cancer most feared by patients, the government and medical authorities. It is the number one killer, both in men and in women. Outside of surgery for very early cases, conventional therapies can offer no help. The ACS projected that in 1999 there would be 171,600 new cases of lung cancer, and 158,900 men and women would die from it.[1]

Fortunately, this is one of the malignancies in which the

metabolic therapy put together by my father more than thirty years ago has been the most successful. In an internal review of more than two hundred patient files, 50 percent of our patients with lung cancer outside the realm of surgery were alive after two years of treatment and 30 percent after five years. You may be surprised that I think these are optimistic figures—only three successes for every ten patients. However, it most definitely is.

Statistics from even the "best" centers in world show that when patients with cancer of the lung are outside the realm of surgery, close to 100 percent die within twelve months, no matter what the therapy, and no patients are alive after five years.[2]

High doses of emulsified vitamin A, given orally in drops, are beneficial in treating cancer of the lung, especially the "squamous cell carcinoma." Possible side effects in highly sensitive patients can include headaches, muscle weakness in the legs or severe dryness of the skin, nose and mouth. If side effects are experienced, we reduce the dosage or suspend treatment for a short period and try again later.

Cancer of the prostate

No other cancer affects men more than cancer of the prostate. The ACS projected that 179,300 men would be diagnosed with prostate cancer in 1999, and 37,000 would die.[3] Fortunately, men tend to die *with* cancer of the prostate rather than *because* of it.

Several reports show that at least 80 percent of men eighty years of age or older who died from causes other than cancer were found to have cancer of the prostate in routinely performed autopsies.[4] In many situations, the patient's quality of life was never affected by it. Even orthodox medicine has a prostate cancer option called "watchful waiting." Unfortunately, very few doctors advise patients of this option; instead, they ruin the patient's good quality of life with aggressive procedures. The results are generally favorable, as far as the cancer goes, but what benefit is it for the patient to be cured but left impotent (66 percent of patients end up impotent after radical prostatectomy) or incontinent (30 percent incidence of incontinence after radical prostatectomy)?[5] Many suffer a combination of both. Why go through the suffering when "living in peace" with a cancerous prostate is a viable option?

Living with prostate cancer is the first option we offer patients whose quality of life has not been affected by this cancer. But we don't just wait for something to happen; we start combating the cancer in a nonaggressive way, offering alternative and effective therapies. But some patients have very aggressive prostate cancer, in which the tumor spreads rapidly and threatens the life of the patient in a short time.

We conducted a clinical study with eight hundred patients who had previously been treated with surgery, radiation and hormone therapies that had "failed" them. These patients had been sent home to die because "there was nothing else to do." (This is the condition in which most of our patients come to us, not only with prostate cancer, but with all cancers.)

Our approach with patients with advanced prostate cancer has consistently given amazing results. After five years, 86 percent of the patients were alive! The common denominator was excellent quality of life. Notice that I said "alive," not cured. Only about 20 percent of those had no tumor activity whatsoever, but the ones with some remnant cancer were as happy as the ones where no tumor was detectable.

We give these patients our metabolic therapy and antiandrogen hormones such as Lupron, Eulexin or Honvan. The side effects can include pain and enlargement of the breasts when taken for a long period of time. If the cancer has metastasized to bones, we add intravenous calcium and aredia. If the bones start to crack or if the patient is suffering extensive bone pain, we recommend radiation to harden the bones and alleviate the pain. Few of our patients have suffered from impotence or incontinence.

Many testimonies of our prostate cancer patients are posted at our website (www.oasisofhope.com). You will enjoy reading the testimony of one of them in Appendix D.

Cancer of the breast

Though the incidence of breast cancer is low in men, it is the cancer most feared by women. The ACS expected that 175,000 women and 1,300 men would be diagnosed with breast cancer in 1999, and 43,300 women and 400 men would die because of it.[6] This cancer has the fastest incidence increase. More has been published about breast cancer than any other malignancy; yet the approved therapies have only helped to prolong life, and that many times at the expense of quality—not only aesthetically, but also physically because of severe side effects.

The treatment of cancer of the breast is extremely complicated because many aspects of women's physiology participate in the tumor's behavior. The same type of tumor has a completely different impact on a woman who is seventy as opposed to a woman who is thirty. The younger the woman, the more aggressive the tumor activity tends to be.

Hormonal aspects of the disease play a definitive role in breast cancer. Surgery has different applications depending on size and location. More and more surgeons around the globe are coming to the conclusion that Crile was right all along (see chapter seven), and lumpectomies and breast-conserving surgery (as we at Oasis have done for the last thirty-six years) have gained acceptance from the medical community. Again, our mode of therapy has given us much encouragement.

When a patient with this disease comes to us, we add to the metabolic therapy anti-estrogen medications like Tamoxifen and Megace, even if the hormone receptors are reported to be negative. These therapies are beneficial because estrogen makes breast cancer grow. A possible side effect is increased appetite, and Megace may provoke fluid retention or blood clots. Our files indicate a 30 percent five-year survival rate.

Dee Simmons is a wonderful example of a victorious breast cancer survivor. You can read her story in Appendix E.

Cancer of the colon with metastasis to the liver

Cancer of the colon is on the increase, and I believe that junk food is responsible for such increase in incidence in the younger generation. The ACS projected that 94,700 people would be diagnosed with colon cancer, and 47,900 would die in the U.S. in 1999.[7] Even though all cancers are related to our eating habits, the relationship of colon cancer to food is extremely close. Just a few years ago this cancer typically occurred in people at retirement age; now it is not uncommon to see the forty-something age group fall prey to it. I have even treated a sixteen-year-old for cancer of the colon!

As with most cancers, early stages can be treated quite efficiently with surgery, and up to 85 percent cure rates can be achieved. But when this cancer spreads to the liver or lungs, the prognosis darkens. It is in this stage that most of our patients come to us.

Liver metastases are the greatest threat to life. We conducted a prospective clinical trial with patients suffering from cancer of the colon with metastasis to the liver with a procedure that I developed, based on other researchers' information. Localized intravenous chemotherapy (5FU) is directed to the liver via a special catheter inserted in a branch of the portal vein. Our results were very encouraging. We were able to offer our patients a 30 percent five-year survival, whereas the possibilities with chemotherapy alone offer a 0 percent survival.

Sometimes we will prescribe oral chemotherapy (Tegafur), especially if 5FU has been used previously and failed. Side effects, such as depletion of white blood cell count or mouth ulcerations, are rare because we use localized therapies or low-to-moderate dose therapies. The results have been impressive.

Read Donald Factor's testimony about his treatment for cancer that had metastasized to the liver; you will find it in Appendix C.

REALISTIC LIFESTYLE CHANGES

APPARENTLY MARK TWAIN had much experience with physicians because he said, "The only way to keep your health is to eat what you don't want, drink what you don't like and do what you'd druther not." But it is very important to make a commitment to health and to the necessary lifestyle changes that promote healing and prevention. I have noticed that patients enthusiastically immerse themselves in dietary programs that are intense, like the Gerson or Malkmus diets, only to cheat continually. But those who comply do well and have something to say "Hallelujah" about. Compliance is paramount.

Each patient's personality must be taken into consideration when recommending therapies and prevention resources. There are Peter-type and Paul-type patients. Some, like the apostle Peter, will have ups and downs in their commitment to a program; others from the onset will not sway an inch, like the apostle Paul.

If a patient with the Peter-type personality frets that "to safeguard one's health at the cost of too strict a diet is a tiresome illness indeed,"[8] then a realistic program should be established for him or her. The benefits and consequences should be laid out, and the patient should be allowed to make his or her own decision.

We encourage our patients to be in charge. They may accept, reject or delay any of our recommendations, but we try to give them sufficient information on which to make intelligent and informed decisions. What I recommend according to my experience may not be in the patient's best interest, because the patient knows his or her body best. A patient who feels that losing any part of his or her anatomy is not acceptable may consciously reject any surgery, thereby accepting whatever outcome. Imposing a specific treatment just because statistically it gives better results is not always the best. Statistics are not necessarily applicable to individuals—singular, unique and wondrously and wonderfully made individuals.

All our medication, remedies, nutritional supplements, vitamins and health-oriented resources are always provided in an environment of hope, faith and love. And the only therapy is that given to all our patients is prayer. No matter how special the needs of a patient may be, prayer is a resource we all can take advantage of.

But the best cure for cancer is prevention. Let's find out how to pursue that course.

10

The Power of Prevention

EVEN THOUGH IT'S a replica, I enjoy it tremendously. With its 300-horse-powered "hot-engine" and a five-speed transmission, my Ford-powered, Jaguar-suspended Cobra race car can elevate some kind of dust. I love speed, and for my personality type, it's therapeutic. Whenever my schedule—or I should say my schedulers—allow, I get in that powerful vintage machine and have some fun in the races with the old-timers—a bunch of gray-haired (the ones who still have hair), good-spirited show-offs who get together to race these big, incredibly beautiful and powerful toys.

But don't think for a moment that we dress up in those fire-resistant suits, put on those helmets, get inside those rollbar-caged cockpits and strap ourselves into those special race-seat harnesses just for a Sunday stroll in the park. No, we get our money's worth from our toys by achieving speeds of up to 130 miles per hour on curvy roads.

People believe that racers have a death wish. Well, I certainly do not. The safety measures I take to avoid accidents are substantial. In fact, once I trained and learned to share the "road" with professionals, I realized how truly dangerous freeways are. The incidence of fatal accidents on racetracks is infinitely lower than that on freeways, roads or streets. That's because race-car drivers not only drive extremely well, but they also take many measures to lower the risks.

MANAGING OUR HEALTH

LOWERING RISKS TO our health increases the length and quality of our lives. Certainly many variables are outside our control, but the responsibility to protect, maintain, cherish and respect our bodies—the single most important asset given to us—is definitely 100 percent ours. When we are also blessed with the gift of good health, the least we should do is to manage our lives in such a way as to reduce the risk of losing it.

I find it sad that because good health is free, many don't appreciate it until it's too late. We are taught from a very young age to value and protect our material assets, but not our good health. We purchase insurance policies to protect our goods, yet even the most comprehensive health insurance policy cannot ensure good health. So, managing risks wisely is the most responsible way to maintain and even to recuperate health.

The optimum way to manage our health is by means of prevention. For many people, prevention means having an annual physical exam. Let's examine that idea.

The annual physical exam

The yearly physical or medical checkup is the premier tool upon which modern society depends for prevention of disease. Although the annual physical may make people feel secure, it can also encourage them to continue with unhealthy lifestyles and can mask long-term problems.

I have been picking on the Americans a lot, so I'll give them a break (for now). The Japan Hospital Association

The Power of Prevention

(JHA) publishes annually a report on the health habits and status of the Japanese people as measured by the number of clean bills of health given in medical checkups. According to their records, in the last fourteen years the "health" of the Japanese, especially those between ages forty and fifty, has steadily declined. In 1984 nearly 30 percent of persons had no "irregularities" in their checkups; in 1998 only 15.8 percent were rewarded with a clean bill of health, "the worst figure on record."

Most of the participants in the medical checkups suffered from hyperglycemia (abnormally high level of glucose in the blood), high cholesterol and triglycerides (high levels of fats in the bloodstream) and obesity.[1] These abnormalities are all precursors to the "Big 5" (the diseases that cause 80 percent of all deaths in the U.S.)—cancer, heart disease, diabetes, obesity and high blood pressure. In Japan, the number one cause of death is already cancer, a trend that most industrialized countries soon will follow.

Of course, the JHA blames the westernized lifestyle of modern Japan, and I could not agree more. Consider the fact that Japan's overall cancer incidence and mortality are the same as those of America. Individual types of cancer may vary, but the absolute per capita numbers are virtually the same.

But at question here is the preventative value of the medical checkup, which relies heavily on blood test results. But blood tests do not necessarily reflect what is going on in the organs at the cellular level; thus they are of limited value. So having all the tests come out within normal range does not necessarily mean that the organs are really healthy.

I see two major problems with medical checkups: 1) Being awarded a clean bill of health can give a patient a false sense of security to continue with a deleterious lifestyle; and 2) the danger of not testing "completely" healthy (an 84 percent chance in Japan) puts a patient at the mercy of the hospital's medical care for blood alterations that do not need medical treatment.

Another problem is the well-known fact that laboratory tests are persistently unreliable. Some patients are "cured" of the suggested disease just by repeating the test! Reports of 40 percent false negative or false positive results are commonly accepted in the industry.[2]

After an annual physical, chances are that a patient will walk out of the hospital or doctor's office with prescription drugs. The medications used for lowering blood sugar and cholesterol have been under scientific attack because, even though they do lower sugar and cholesterol, they have not been proven to prolong a patient's life. In fact, when these drugs were tested in long-term double blind studies, the patients who took the placebos (sugar pills, of all things!) lived longer, even with their elevated levels of glucose and cholesterol.[3]

But it's not all bad news. Understanding the limitations of a physical will help you to guard yourself from the mirage while taking advantage of the benefits. If you choose to visit your doctor regularly for preventative measures, you may be able to monitor the changes your body experiences due to your efforts to improve lifestyle. Cardiovascular evaluation may show you if you are in bad shape, and it may encourage you to do something to improve your physical conditioning as well as your heart and lung function.

Most importantly, a medical checkup may detect diseases in early stages that can be helped. However, let's think about this concept a little.

Early detection—or prevention?

In a truly masterful marketing strategy, the medical industry, especially oncologists, introduced decades ago an idea that gained universal acceptance: *Prevention is early detection.*

The Power of Prevention

There is no doubt that many diseases, even cancer, when found in early stages can be better treated, sometimes even cured. Cancer of the colon found in early stages has a cure rate of up to 85 percent with surgery.[4] One of the values of the Pap smear is that cervical cancer can be detected in its early stages, at which time surgery is curative in up to 99 percent of the cases. Yes, cancer may be prevented, but the fact remains that these and all other tests detect an illness or a malfunction *after the fact.* They do not prevent the disease from coming in the first place.

By definition, stopping the development of illness is the sole purpose of prevention. Everything else is cutting your losses, even if your losses are small because you were able to detect your disease early. In the case of cancer, the established orthodox medical system has not been able either to protect people from cancer or to effectively treat it. So, health authorities cleverly packaged the generally accepted concept that early detection is prevention. Funny, isn't it? Because in reality, no matter how early cancer is detected, if it is present at all, it wasn't prevented.

Some actual preventative measures are offered in the medical system, but they are either extremely meager and given without conviction, or they are extremely radical and offered coercively. For instance, dietary changes are proffered in most of the medical associations (cancer, arthritis, diabetes), but in practice, no real efforts are spent with patients to educate them about nutrition. This type of approach has been proven ineffectual over and over. Additionally, chemotherapy is offered as a preventative measure, and many patients who fear cancer are undergoing this paradoxical measure, when most, if not all, chemotherapeutic agents are carcinogenic!

Applications from genetics are starting to find their way into preventative medical practice. One of which is the idea that if a person has a high risk of developing cancer at a nonvital target site, removing the target organ would prevent that patient from developing the cancer. Such is the case with breast cancer.

Young women, usually in their late teens or early forties with a "strong family history" of breast cancer (two or more first-degree relatives with cancer of the breast) and the presence of one or both of the breast cancer genes (BRCA1 or BRCA2), are considered high risk and candidates for prophylactic (preventative) mastectomies. In other words, doctors remove a healthy breast in order to prevent the possibility of the woman getting breast cancer.

I am dumbfounded by the fact that people, much less doctors, could come up with such a Machiavellian preventative measure. Only the incalculable persuasive power of fear can coerce women to be disfigured willingly, believing in a prophylactic procedure that makes such little sense.

If we scratch the feeble surface of the breakthrough ideas of genetics, their impact on health becomes highly questionable. The United States has one of the highest incidences of breast cancer in the world, close to 100 cases per 100,000.[5] China, on the other hand, has the lowest—around 1 per 100,000. According to the genetic theorem, this would mean that Americans have a heavy cancer-of-the-breast genetic load and the Chinese do not.

Why is it, then, that when the Chinese emigrate to the States, those who adopt the American lifestyle acquire the same incidence for breast cancer as the Americans? Yet those who maintain their traditional eating habits maintain a low incidence of cancer of the breast. Much ink has been used writing on this subject. Instead of searching for malevolent genes, let's look for family cookbooks and destroy them!

I do not believe that genetics offers the sought-after magic answer. We are waiting for the scientific solution, and there is none. Preventing cancer involves lifestyle changes.

The Power of Prevention

At the beginning of this new century, people put their hope for health in medical science and technology, believing that's where the silver bullet will be found. Meanwhile, they are only marginally (and for the most part erroneously) educated about what to do to fend off the most common killer diseases.

GOOD HEALTH—A MATTER OF PUBLIC POLICY

IN MARCH 1997 I was invited to speak in the United States before the House of Representatives of the State of Georgia. The House was discussing the options available to lower health care costs for the elderly in nursing homes. Most of the ideas concerned providing services, such as on-site nursing, on-site doctors' visits and purchasing diagnostic equipment vs. outsourcing lab work. But one of the representatives had read my book, *Health in the 21st Century, Will Doctors Survive?*, and thought that my message would help the task force focus on the wellness of the elderly rather than on their diseases.

The honor and responsibility of being there rested heavily on my shoulders. I felt uneasy (terrified!) because I have been openly critical of the government for being so "benevolent" in permitting the chemical and food industries to pollute our world and our foods. Although not all the representatives were happy about my visit, I could not pass up an opportunity like that to say what was on my heart.

"Health is not a medical problem; disease is," I told them. "Health is primarily a political issue." At this, some of them looked up from their notes (or novels, who knows? Maybe they have learned something from the Mexican politicians!) and gave me a surprised look. "This is not new," I continued. "A politician (and prophet) three thousand years ago said it better than anybody I know: 'My people perish for lack of knowledge.'"

"What *is* new," I paused for a bit of dramatic effect, "is that

165

you invited a Mexican quack, from Tijuana, of all places, to show you the way to lower healthcare costs in this great State of Georgia! You must be desperate!" The ensuing laughter broke the ice, and I had the opportunity to talk to people who could really make a difference in the health of society.

I told them that the policy to make wearing seat belts obligatory was right on the money because it saves lives. Yet the policy to allow cigarettes to be sold kills. Policy either promotes or discourages good health. The medical industry in a very clever way has usurped this responsibility from our lawmakers, and the lawmakers have been happy to acquiesce. This shift has impacted communal health in developed countries as well as in the Third World. I let them know that balance between progress and well-being remains the lawmakers' responsibility.

The cost of healthcare is a major concern in the United States, so the government has sponsored a number of studies to assess risk factors and find cost-effective solutions. I told the Georgia representatives that these studies concluded that the previous dietary concepts embraced by science, industry and policy have been wrong and costly in the worst kind of way—people are paying for them with their lives. The five major killer diseases of developed countries have all been unequivocally linked to lifestyle and the Standard American Diet (appropriately abbreviated SAD).

I also let them know what D. M. Hegsted, M.D., professor of nutrition at the Harvard School of Public Health, said to the United States Senate Select Committee on Nutrition and Human Needs. He was speaking on the study *Dietary Goals for the United States,* which strongly associated dietary habits of the American population to chronic degenerative diseases. It should be emphasized that this Standard American Diet, which affluent people generally consume, is everywhere associated with a similar disease pattern—high rates of ischemic heart disease, certain forms of cancer, diabetes and obesity.

> They are epidemic in our population. We cannot afford
> to temporize. We have an obligation to inform the
> public of the current state of knowledge and to assist
> the public in making the correct food choices. To do less
> is to avoid our responsibility.[6]

After all the facts were in, the chairman of the U.S. Senate
Select Committee on Nutrition and Human Needs concluded, "The purpose of this report is to point out that the
eating patterns of this century represent as critical a public
concern as any now before us."[7]

"Powerful words, don't you think?" I asked the representatives. "But wait—there is more." I went on to tell them
that the chairman of this committee called the Senate and
every other pertinent authority to action in no uncertain
terms: "Those of us within government have an obligation to
acknowledge this. The public wants some guidance, wants to
know the truth, and hopefully today we can lay the corner-
stone for the building of better health for all Americans
through better nutrition."[8]

Then I let the bomb drop. "The problem is that these feel-
good words were pronounced by Senator George McGovern on
January 14, 1977. More than twenty years later, Americans
continue eating themselves to death. We Mexicans have made a
name for ourselves with our *mañana* ("I'll do it tomorrow")
culture, but I think the American lawmakers have outdone us
on this one."

Before my visit to the House of Representatives, I had
contacted one of the more plush retirement homes in the
Georgia city of Warner Robins and requested their menu.
They assured me that expert dieticians and nutritionists
approved this menu and that the medical staff had agreed
that it was a healthy, nutritious diet. Here it is:

The Hope of Living Cancer Free

BREAKFAST	LUNCH	DINNER
Cereal/choice	Fish	Bar-B-Q pork
Egg as desired	French fries	Baked beans
Sausage	Coleslaw	Sliced tomatoes
Biscuit	Fiesta cornbread	Bun
Margarine	Lemon pudding	Peaches
Jelly	Tea/coffee	Milk
Milk		Tea/coffee
Coffee	Garnish: Ketchup	Garnish: Pickle slice

I was shocked that the only healthy food in the whole day's menu was the sliced tomatoes. The eggs were substitute eggs, and the peaches were canned—and those were the healthier items!

I encouraged the representatives in Georgia not to procrastinate any longer. I suggested some guidelines for health policy for the elderly, which included implementation of healthy diets in the nursing homes, education, providing vitamin and mineral supplementation, exercise programs and taking advantage of their wisdom rather than making them feel useless. If they implemented this type of policy, I remarked, they would be rewarded very soon with happier seniors who would contribute tax dollars rather than use them up.

The society's well-being is inseparable from the society's physical and emotional health. Order and well-being in a society depend on the policies established by the government. Therefore, good health is fundamentally a public policy issue.

THE STRUGGLE FOR DIETARY GUIDELINES

SO, WHAT HAPPENED in the U.S. Senate after they discovered that the Standard American Diet was killing us? Before establishing any policy, the congressmen conferred with experts in the field, namely the American Medical Association (AMA) and the American Dietetic Association (ADA), regarding the results of the report.

The ADA responded in a decisive letter to Senator McGovern's Select Committee on Nutrition and Human Needs, which included this comment: "An analysis of these meals will quickly reveal that they are so poor nutritionally, they would contribute more to a person remaining in the hospital than helping them get well and be able to return to their homes."[9]

The AMA was not for the policy either, stating firmly that the dietary changes recommended were scientifically unfounded. They suggested further study on the matter: "The evidence for assuming that benefits to be derived from the adoption of such universal goals as set forth in the report is not conclusive and...potential for harmful effects...would occur through adoptions of the proposed national goals."[10]

After reading these responses, I wondered what kind of unreasonable dietetic recommendations the report made to create such a strong response from the health experts. Let's see the guidelines to decide for ourselves.

* Increase vegetables, fruits and grains
* Increase fiber
* Decrease total and saturated fat
* Leaner meats and low-fat dairy products
* Decrease cholesterol
* Decrease salt and sugar
* Use healthy methods to prepare food[11]

It boggles my mind that health experts would go on record stating that these dietary measures would be harmful.

The AMA wanted more epidemiological research because, they argued, the scientific method must establish the specific relationship between dietary habits and chronic disease in order for them to acknowledge it. Since the overwhelming data in the report put the blame on dietary fat intake, they wanted to see proof of the specific pathway by which fat caused disease.

Indeed, the politicians were so impressed by the profoundness of the experts' request that more money was diverted to continue looking into the epidemiological causes of the increase in chronic degenerative illnesses.

Over the next years, report followed report, all saying that the Standard American Diet (SAD) was the culprit for much of the cardiovascular disease, cancer, diabetes, obesity and high blood pressure.[12] Five years later a most definitive project came to press, titled *Dietary Guidelines for Americans.*[13] This report agreed with the others, but it introduced the fact that the environment also played an important role increasing the incidence of chronic disease.

The congressmen are not entirely to blame, but I do believe that they conveniently washed their hands of it, resting the case on the pillars of science. This diffused a complex issue that would economically affect two of the most profitable industries in the country—the food industry and the medical industry.

In 1989 the most comprehensive of all the epidemiological reports, *The Surgeon General's Report on Nutrition and Health,*[14] came out. Former Surgeon General C. Everett Koop, M.D., Sc.D., concluded that the most important recommendation "is to reduce dietary fat.... This advice is not new. But it is now substantiated."

The report can be summarized in three points:

- Improvements in diet can reduce risk of chronic disease.
- Similar dietary recommendations apply to virtually all chronic diseases.
- Reduction of fat intake is the first dietary priority.

One of the most ambitious epidemiological research projects

ever to take place has been going on now for more than fifteen years in China. A multinational group consisting of members from the United States (Cornell University), the United Kingdom (Oxford) and the government of China have been cooperating to gather information. The China Project is researching many aspects of disease, one of which is diet (especially its relationship with cancer.[15]

This study confirms that the amount of fat and protein ingested is directly related to the incidence of cancer, especially cancer of the breast. As mentioned before, the Chinese have one of the lowest, if not the lowest, incidence of cancer of the breast. They consume about four grams of animal protein per day. In other words, it would take a Chinese woman about one hundred days to consume one pound of animal protein (meats and dairy).

In the West, of course, consuming a pound a day of animal protein would not be unheard of. But the average incidence of cancer of the breast in Western women is about 100 cases per 100,000.

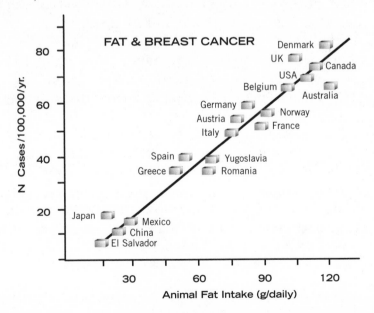

There is a close relationship between fat consumption and breast cancer. In Germany, Austria, France, Norway and other countries where fat consumption is around 90 grams a day, the incidence is 50 to 70 cases per 100,000. Spanish, Romanian and Greek women normally ingest less than 65 grams of fat per day, and their incidence of breast cancer is between 30 and 40 cases per 100,000. In underdeveloped countries like El Salvador, Mexico, China, along with developed countries that choose to eat low fat diets, such as the Japanese, fat consumption is between 20 and 30 grams a day, and the incidence of cancer of the breast drops to between 1 to 20 cases per 100,000.

The major sources of saturated fat in the current United States food supply (the Standard American Diet) are:[16]

- Meat (35 percent of the total saturated fat available)
- Dairy products (20 percent)
- Cooking and table fats and oils (34 percent)

Former Surgeon General C. Everett Koop's 1989 report revealed that "the average amount of saturated fat in the American diet has not changed for more than 50 years."[17] Add another decade to that statement. "More than 40 percent of Americans eat no fruit on any given day, 50 percent eat no vegetables other than potatoes, beans or salad, and more than 80 percent eat no high-fiber bread or cereal."[18]

As these reports were being brought to the attention of the media, the information started trickling down to the public and to the food industry. The "scandalous" recommendations of the late seventies were now slowly becoming "common sense" to most people. Still, no real policy action was or has been established to resolve the issue.

The Power of Prevention

THE ROLE OF THE FOOD INDUSTRY

WHAT BEGAN AS a crusade to change dietary habits to improve the health of the nation and the world (because many countries follow the lead America sets) turned into a marketing opportunity for the food industry. Thousands of new food products were introduced into the marketplace. Of these, a large percentage were candy, gum or snacks. The producers of food, candy, soft drinks, fast foods, beer, wine and liquor were among the top one hundred of the companies of the Fortune 500.

Of course, the industry was quick to acknowledge that saturated fat was deadly, so they introduced margarine (which doctors rapidly endorsed). The words *light* and *healthy* were introduced to fight the fat threat, and products with these words on their labels have increased sales *even though they are often neither light nor healthy.* Processed foods make money for the food industry, but they don't lead to good health.

The consumer wants healthy junk food, but it doesn't exist. So the sick feel sicker when they are told what they should eat the rest of their lives!

We all know that eating is much more than a way to please our taste buds or an occasion to socialize. Both of these are important indeed, but the basic purpose for eating is to provide our organisms with the fuel they require to function properly.

One of the problems of our modern world is that some have no money to buy food and the rest have too much and eat too much. The hi-tech foods of today have an abundance of calories with few nutrients, if any. The most prevalent complication of such an overfed and undernourished society is obesity.

This problem has affected our communities in more than

173

the obvious ways. Yankee Stadium was built in 1922, and in 1978 the owners had to rebuild it in order to accommodate our more modern shapes. The contractors increased the width of the seats from twenty inches to twenty-four inches. Not only did the reconstruction cost the owners millions of dollars, but they also lost eight thousand seats!

In the age range of fifty-five to sixty-five, just under half—48.7 percent—of Americans are obese.[19] Each year three hundred thousand U.S. citizens die from obesity. It is difficult to blame them when the exposure to such foods is so overwhelming.

The original preventative purpose of these studies— good health through prevention—succumbed to the claws of the economy-driven society, including the food and health industries. But the preventative power of the information has not been lost completely. Many of us gained information, and it is not too late to multiply efforts to share practical preventative measures with those who understand that lifestyle changes are the best and cheapest way to add years to our lives and life to our years.

Do not let "scientific proof" sway you away from common sense. Resist falling into the belief that it just doesn't make any difference what we do or do not do. This apocalyptic mentality dooms people just to wait for pollution or wars or disease to catch up with them and destroy them.

Every little thing you do does make a difference. Providing food for the hungry in your area will definitely not solve the problem of world hunger, but it will make a difference to that one child or that one family who, because you cared, had something to eat that night before going to sleep. Being overwhelmed is understandable, but conveniently feeling defeated before you even start is irresponsible. Choosing to be responsible will always make a good, solid, meaningful difference in your life.

SEVEN HEALTHY HABITS

I HAVE LED you through the bumpy road of preventative choices. If we want to really be free of the plague of cancer, we must teach our children and their children to adopt a healthy lifestyle and an activist mentality.

If the following suggestions seem overwhelming, narrow them down as much as needed to make them practical for you. Perhaps you will decide that becoming a vegetarian is the most responsible choice, yet it is a practical and emotional impossibility for you, plus it would lead to suicidal tendencies! In that case, I recommend that you set more down-to-earth objectives. Do what you can. Then, step by step, who knows?

Here are my seven habits of successful health risk managers:

1. Wear seat belts.

This won't prevent you from getting cancer, but even cancer patients can lose fingers or legs in an accident. Honor life and body parts; they are still not replaceable. Use helmets and all the pads designed to protect your body when you enjoy a sport or a hobby.

2. Stop smoking, and stop drinking alcohol.

I have not wasted much time so far in this "no-brainer" preventative measure. Do not ingest or inject any substance that will deteriorate your body's capabilities. The only exception could be a *small* glass of red wine with lunch or dinner. This amount can have beneficial effects.

3. Exercise.

Use your body to its maximum potential. If you do not, it will deteriorate faster. Movement will give you strength and agility into your retirement years. Plus, exercise diminishes the incidence of the "Big 5."

4. Forget the Standard American Diet (SAD).

Consume only the best. Follow the recommended dietary suggestions in this book. Many studies substantiate the preventative and curative possibilities of a good diet. Remember to set reachable goals.

You only live once. Demand organically grown foods. Eat only free-range meats if you eat meat. Avoid processed and precooked foods. Supplement with vitamins, minerals, enzymes, phytochemicals and fiber because, due to pollution and overuse of the land, even organically grown foods do not have all the nutrients our bodies need for optimum performance.

5. Participate in making the future better.

Become an activist for change. Your personal contribution, no matter how small, makes an enormous difference. Put pressure on government to stop protecting an industry that is poisoning us, and with your dollars, support businesses that provide good, wholesome food. In order for our air and everything else our bodies need to become cleaner and purer, participate actively in making constructive changes in our environment. Leave a better world for the next generation.

6. Have a annual or semiannual physical.

Take advantage of the information you receive, and resolve the problems in the most sensible and natural way. Plus, early detection of a problem could save your life.

7. Get medical insurance.

Medical insurance is extremely valuable for acute care. Some policies cover alternative therapies. One of those would offer you the best coverage.

Evaluate all the information, digest it and then take action. The choice is yours. If our policymakers do not establish positive health policies and if the medical industry continues with only the intervention approach, then it is up to you and me to establish personal and family preventative policies.

God gave these words to Moses to present to the Israelite people. But they also apply to us today.

> I call heaven and earth as witnesses today against you, that I have set before you life and death, blessing and cursing; therefore choose life, that both you and your descendants may live.
>
> —DEUTERONOMY 30:19, NKJV

Section III:
Restoration From Above

11

Why Do Bad Things Happen to Good People?

WHEN I WAS a young man, my sister Estela, only thirty-six years old, was killed in a plane crash. She was a Spirit-filled, born-again Christian, a schoolteacher, a pastor's wife and a mother of two young children. I remember the joy of the Lord that she shared with so many people and all of the people whom she personally brought closer to Christ. She was in the prime of a fruitful life and ministry when suddenly it ended.

When the candle of life is snuffed without explanation, most ask: Why her? Why me? Why now? Why not to a "bad" person instead? Why cancer? These questions are extremely difficult to answer; perhaps we won't really understand until we enter eternity. But at the heart of all these questions is God—the One who is at the end of our desperate search for answers.

Most cultures, regardless of their beliefs, regard a higher entity (God, gods, the absolute, Mother Nature, "the man upstairs") as the giver or taker of life. However, in our modern society, faith in science has taken the place of faith in God.

Science says our existence is a mishap, a random event that happened sometime after the big bang billions of years ago. Life and all of its forms have evolved since then, they say. This proposition seems more scientifically sound and soothing to our rational minds than is the idea of a Creator. The problem I have with evolution is that at its core, it is no different than any other theological position. It relies on faith.

Everyone knows that it takes faith to make sense of Christ and Christianity. Yet, as a Christian, I envy the faith of those who believe in evolution, because my faith is limited to believing in God as the Creator. Those who believe in evolution have to have faith that the human body, with its one hundred trillion cells all working in harmony, plus the vast universe, all happened by chance. Now, that takes a whole lot more faith than I have! I'll stick with creation.

WHY IS THERE DISEASE?

SCIENCE DOES NOT, by any stretch of the imagination, explain all that is going on in this world. The deep questions within us cannot be answered by science. Even the issues of sickness and health must be addressed from a spiritual dimension as well as a scientific aspect. Science, evolution and all their theories just don't resolve the profound issues we face.

Creationists believe there was a time when perfect balance existed between the Creator and creation, a time of perfect health with no sickness. Adam and Eve enjoyed the cleanest, most unpolluted environment ever in Eden. Disease and death did not threaten their perfect balance with their environment. As long as those conditions existed, disease could not exist. We can draw the logical conclusion that humans were designed to live forever.

What happened? In my opinion, in the instant that they ate of the forbidden fruit, the perfect balance between Creator and creation was lost, broken by sin. At that moment a dramatic paradigm shift occurred—the path to death was opened in both the physical world and the spiritual world.

Now, instead of being born to live forever, we are born, we grow, we reproduce ourselves and we die. Sin disrupted the perfect balance between God and man, and it opened the door for illness to rush in. The Bible clearly teaches that the wages of sin is death, and death is directly linked to the slow loss of health (sickness).

This biblical concept of illness and death may seem harsh, but it is not unique. Many religions, even those not influenced by Judaism, have spiritual rituals for healing that incorporate asking for forgiveness for any transgressions that may have brought the disease upon them. It seems that deep inside we know that sickness is unnatural; it's not the way God intended it. And we know that something must bring on sickness. The question is, What?

SICKNESS IS NONDISCRIMINATING

SOME MAY SAY that all disease is the consequence of personal sin, but that is obviously not the case. If we unknowingly eat contaminated food, most likely we will visit the toilet many times during the night because that famous balance was broken. So all sickness is not caused by personal sin.

I have heard gentle Christian people and well-meaning pastors say to the sick, "Confess your sins, and you will be made whole again." Others who are more aggressive tell the sick that because they have hidden sin, they have brought the illness upon themselves.

I have noticed that when some of these same pastors get sick themselves, they change their positions. But I have a lot of compassion for these people. Humility is a great teacher; it has taught me not to cast stones at others, but instead to come alongside them and see how the Lord can use me to help them up.

Jesus clearly taught His disciples that disease was not always due to sin. When they came across a blind man, His disciples asked:

> Master, who did sin, this man, or his parents, that he was born blind? Jesus answered, Neither hath this man sinned, nor his parents: but that the works of God should be made manifest in him.
>
> —JOHN 9:2–3

Jesus did not blame this man—or his parents—for his blindness. He indicated there was a higher purpose for it.

I believe that sickness, released into the world through sin, is nondiscriminating. In other words, it brought disequilibrium to everybody. It's like a chemical plant that disposes of its toxic waste into the river—the whole community is affected. Disease will eventually affect all of us. Did you know that there are no natural causes of death? Even with an accident, death is caused by a break of the perfect balance—in that case, an instant breakdown. A breaking of this balance is always the cause of death.

PURPOSES AND REASONS FOR DISEASE

WE ONLY HAVE to walk out to get the morning paper or turn on the television to see that there is great sorrow, tragedy and decay in our world. Though it wasn't originally designed that way, it's that way for now, and disease is part of that. However, the way in which we respond to disease is what is most important.

Chastisement

Some diseases were brought upon man directly by God for a specific reason. This is not a popular belief in today's Christian circles, but it is biblical.

Why Do Bad Things Happen to Good People?

Who can forget God's dramatic reaction against Aaron and Miriam for opposing Moses?

> And the anger of the Lord was kindled against them; and he departed. And the cloud departed from off the tabernacle; and, behold, Miriam became leprous, white as snow: and Aaron looked upon Miriam, and, behold, she was leprous.
>
> —Numbers 12:9–10

Nothing is more displeasing to God than disobedience. God's chosen people, Israel, again and again tested God's tolerance with disobedience until He responded.

> If you do not carefully follow all the words of this law, which are written in this book, and do not revere this glorious and awesome name—the Lord your God—the Lord will send fearful plagues on you and your descendants, harsh and prolonged disasters, and severe and lingering illnesses. He will bring upon you all the diseases of Egypt that you dreaded, and they will cling to you.
>
> —Deuteronomy 28:58–60, NIV

> The Lord will strike you with wasting disease, with fever and inflammation, with scorching heat and drought, with blight and mildew, which will plague you until you perish.
>
> —Deuteronomy 28:22, NIV

Unfortunately, the chastisement for their disobedience not only affected them, but the rest of us as well! Plagues were introduced into the world, and they are at work today. They didn't go away. Unfortunately, generations later we still suffer from them.

They will be a sign and a wonder to you and your descendants forever.
—DEUTERONOMY 28:46, NIV

So we have inherited diseases that cannot be avoided, either through prevention or treatment. As a consequence, these terrible plagues are present today and will be with us until Jesus comes again.

A greater purpose

Diseases can be used by God to protect us from greater evils. For instance, we may fall ill and miss an airplane that later crashes. In this way, we were saved by God's use of the sickness.

The apostle Paul was in jeopardy of losing his eternal life in heaven by falling prey to self-assuredness and pride. But God allowed an illness to keep him from committing these arrogant, dangerous sins.

And lest I should be exalted above measure through the abundance of the revelations, there was given to me a thorn in the flesh, the messenger of Satan to buffet me, lest I should be exalted above measure. For this thing I besought the Lord thrice, that it might depart from me. And he said unto me, My grace is sufficient for thee: for my strength is made perfect in weakness.
—2 CORINTHIANS 12:7–9

Our choices

Diseases for chastisement or for a greater purpose are the exception and the extreme. In my opinion, the vast majority of health problems are directly related to the choices we make in our everyday lives through conscious or unconscious carelessness. Even inheritance is not to blame in these.

Why Do Bad Things Happen to Good People?

> I call heaven and earth to record this day against you,
> that I have set before you *life* and *death,* blessing and
> cursing: therefore choose *life,* that both thou and thy
> seed may live.
> —DEUTERONOMY 30:19, EMPHASIS ADDED

Both eternal salvation and earthly quality of life, for the most part, are a matter of choice. We can choose to follow or reject Christ. We can choose to protect or jeopardize our health. Let me explain.

Do you put on seat belts and drive safely? Do you exercise and keep in shape? Do you eat a nutritious diet and maintain a healthy weight, or do you pray that the junk food you continually eat will not harm you and make you fat?

These and other factors determine the health of our society. Cardiovascular diseases, cancer, obesity, diabetes and high blood pressure are the five major killers in developed countries. All these ailments are directly related to poor diet and lack of exercise. Lifestyle affects Christian and non-Christian organisms the same.

By abiding by sound dietary principles, we can reduce—I repeat, reduce—the risk of illness, but we cannot exterminate disease altogether.

WHY ME?

HINDSIGHT, WITHOUT QUESTION, is always 20/20. But how do we deal with the present pain of a disease like cancer and the uncertainty of the immediate future? My heart aches for the dear people who ask the question, "Why me? Why not the serial killer who has been on death row for a couple of decades?"

Recently I was on a radio program being interviewed about prayer in medicine. I received many calls praising the fact that, as a doctor, I was promoting prayer in medical practice. But one hurting caller blurted out, "Yeah, but try praying to a God who gave you a child, an only child, with cerebral palsy." Then he hung up.

A number of my patients have asked me to explain why illness struck them. They tell me how they have led a relatively stress-free life, kept God's commandments, ate right and exercised. Then, if those patients die, the loved ones ask why it happened if the Bible promises healing.

When a person asks over and over again, "Why me, why me, why me?" a wedge between that individual and God occurs because the person's eyes move off God and onto self. If he or she insists on asking this question, and no answer comes, then doubt sets in, which can be followed by anger and even hatred toward God.

At this point, physical cancer can cross over into the spiritual realm and become cancer of the soul. Whether Satan is the father of cancer or not, whether you believe in heaven or not, the ultimate outcome of this kind of desperation will be acquiring spiritually cancerous thoughts of doubt, anger and hatred toward our Maker. I believe that cancer gains the ultimate victory when the physical tumor is able to spread to the soul. Then death abides in the patient even if he is among the living.

If John F. Kennedy were writing this book with me, he might challenge us today by saying, "Ask not, 'Why me?' but, 'Why not me?'" What is so unique about us that we should receive only the good and not the bad? How would we experience the beauty of life if tragedy didn't show it off? Do we have the fortitude to welcome whatever is in store for us and be grateful? It is not whether or not we get sick; it is how we deal with the illness that counts.

The apostle Peter wrote to us, "Dear friends, do not be surprised at the painful trial you are suffering, as though something strange were happening to you" (1 Pet. 4:12, NIV).

Peter was talking about persecution for following Christ, but his instructions reveal that Christians are not shielded 100 percent from suffering or pain.

Job had some "friends" much like the "friends" you might have. They came to mourn with him when he lost all his children and all his possessions at one time. In an effort to explain this great catastrophe, Job's friends told him that he had brought the disaster upon himself, that God had abandoned him. Job's wife even complained about his loyalty to a God who allowed such destruction. But Job wisely responded, "What? shall we receive good at the hand of God, and shall we not receive evil?" (Job 2:10).

Many of my elderly patients recover while the younger ones do not because the elderly more readily take on the attitude "Whatever God wants to do is fine with me." This attitude frees them completely of stress. The younger patients, however, are frequently filled with desperation to live, and the stress of their fight for life turns out to be counterproductive.

Helping my patients transition from fear and doubt to freedom and trust is one of my treatment goals. They are not free and victorious if they are healed of cancer but continue to fear it. I help them redefine victory over cancer. It is not *whether* they live or die; it is *how* they live out the days that God gives them on earth. If we can keep focused on that, we will have victory.

Physical healing is always temporary. Every human being who has ever lived is in the process of dying or has already died. True and permanent healing happens only when we are in perfect balance with the Creator and the rest of creation, and that will not happen here on earth, but in that infinite place some of us call heaven. There and then health will be eternal.

There is more to disease than just getting cured. Dare we

look beneath the surface and see if any hidden treasures lie there?

SUFFERING

THE BIBLE TELLS us that if we love the Lord, everything that happens to us is for our own good. (See Romans 8:28.) How is suffering from an illness of any benefit? If I had a clear answer to that, I would be astonishingly enlightened. A simple experience with my first daughter provided a glimpse into God's wisdom vs. our foolishness and near-sightedness.

At eight months, my daughter was getting squirmy and impatient with getting her diaper changed. As I was struggled with the diaper—all the while fighting the odor and the sheer volume of the toxic waste—she was determined to do a hands-on exploration of the diaper's contents. Just at the moment when she was less than an inch away from it all, I caught her beautiful little hand. I felt heroic—what a catch, and just in the nick of time! But not only was she unappreciative, she was downright angry at me.

At that moment, I felt, in a microcosmic way, what God must feel when He tries to save us from trouble. We believe He is interfering with what we think is best for us.

For many, it is difficult to understand how a God of love can allow His children to experience disease.

> See now that I, even I, am he, and there is no god with me: I kill, and I make alive; I wound, and I heal: neither is there any that can deliver out of my hand.
> —DEUTERONOMY 32:39

When tragedy strikes, sometimes we don't see the good in it, much less comply with the commandment that we should thank God in all that happens to us (1 Thess. 5:18). If we don't understand that God is in charge, we experience only desperation and loss.

The apostle Paul said, "For now we see through glass darkly, but then face to face" (1 Cor. 13:12). Someday, when we are in His presence—if it even matters any more—we will see clearly the blessings that our trials and tribulations brought to us and others. I also believe our eyes will be opened to the tragedies that we avoided through God's unseen intervention.

THE ETERNAL PERSPECTIVE

NO FORMULAS CAN contain the vastness of God. His will is something that *will* be accomplished because He knows what is best for us eternally, not just for the present. If in the present we must suffer as the disciples did, then we must also set our eyes on the glory to come. Nevertheless, we can always resort to the infinite mercy of God.

> Let us therefore come boldly unto the throne of grace, that we may obtain mercy, and find grace to help in time of need.
> —HEBREWS 4:16

> I will heal their backsliding, I will love them freely: for mine anger is turned away from him.
> —HOSEA 14:4

> But God, who is rich in *mercy,* for his great love...For by *grace* are ye saved through faith; and that not of yourselves: it is the *gift* of God: not of works, lest any man should boast.
> —EPHESIANS 2:4, 8–9, EMPHASIS ADDED

It is this mercy that I seek and humbly ask every day for

my personal life and for my patients. God has blessed us at Oasis of Hope Hospital, where we experience miracle after miracle of the grace of God.

But many times we are not satisfied with the mercy God offers. Instead we demand that the grace of God align with our expectations. Don't forget what happened to the Jews after God released them from the oppression of Egypt. God provided them with a cloud that protected them from the sun, a pillar of light to illuminate their nights and manna to eat so that they didn't have to worry about food. But they were not grateful. They missed the variety of the food, especially the meat that they had back in captivity in Egypt (a lot of us would, too!). So the Lord, rather humorously, acquiesced to their demands by giving them flesh to eat—abundantly!

> Ye shall not eat one day, nor two days, nor five days, neither ten days, nor twenty days; but even a whole month, until it come out at your nostrils, and it be loathsome unto you: because that ye have despised the LORD which is among you, and have wept before him, saying, Why came we forth out of Egypt?
> —NUMBERS 11:19–20

Be careful with your demands to the Lord of lords. He is the I AM; He is absolutely sovereign. Only when we are willing to see the greater picture, the eternal perspective, can we understand the enormity of God's grace in sending His only Son to die for our sins that we may live eternally in heaven. Once that truly sinks in, we can be victorious against disease and anything else because we know God is in control, always doing what is best for us.

I will beg for mercy in the time of need, but I will accept His response—either way—as the perfect solution. In this, I will learn something of God's healing ways.

12

God's Healing Ways

SICKNESS CAN BE a powerful motivator or a great discourager. In my life as a physician I have, in a very short time, gone from the exhilaration of a newfound method of treatment to the deflation of defeat at the side of a patient who died before my eyes.

The more experience I gather from my own state of health and that of my patients, the more I'm convinced that ignorance kills. But knowledge is, in general, a powerful preventative force.

Because of that, no one is more privileged than the person who has access to truth. We live in a time of this privilege, not because of the technological advances that make our existence so comfortable, but because we have the Bible, God's Word. In it is the wonderful knowledge of Christ's power of salvation so we would not perish.

WHY AREN'T BELIEVERS HEALTHY?

YES, THOSE WHO believe in Christ are privileged people indeed. But the salvation of our souls has not yet translated into healthy bodies. Statistically, we are as sick or sicker than those who have not accepted—or who have even rejected—Christ as their Savior! What happened to Jesus' promise: "I am come that they might have life, and that they might have it more abundantly" (John 10:10)?

In my practice I see patients who have given their lives to the Lord, who consistently preach the gospel of salvation, yet who still end up losing the war against cancer, heart disease, diabetes and other diseases. To a Christian and a doctor, this is quite discouraging. Young and old, men and women, lay people and clergy—no matter how committed—still succumb to disease. So we must ask, Can we establish a biblical formula to combat disease?

PROMISES OF HEALING

THE BIBLE ABOUNDS with promises about the healing power of God and His wish for us to be healthy.

> But he was wounded for our transgressions, he was bruised for our iniquities: the chastisement of our peace was upon him; and with his stripes we are healed.
> —ISAIAH 53:5

The capability for healing has been extended to us through Jesus Christ and the Holy Ghost.

> And he ordained twelve, that they should be with him, and that he might send them forth to preach, and to have power to heal sicknesses, and to cast out devils.
> —MARK 3:14–15

So it seems as if Christians should not be sick. And if they do fall ill, it seems that perhaps doctors should not be sought; rather, the promises of healing should be sufficient to make the person well. Is that right?

A NUMBER OF ministerial movements have arisen that claim to have infallible formulas for perfect health based upon biblical promises about healing. According to these people, when these formulas fail, it is because of the lack of faith of the patient, the inability of the patient to allow God to work or the presence of demonic forces that the patient is unwilling to release. Although I agree that these and other factors interfere in the work that God can do, I also feel that it's a bit arrogant to believe we can box God into a determined faith formula.

There is no doubt that faith is an important ingredient in many healings in the Bible. We think of the immovable faith of the woman of Canaan who refused to give up without her daughter being healed (Matt. 15:28). It is easy to conclude, then, that faith such as hers is needed for conquering disease; if one doesn't have that faith, then healing will not come. But that is not necessarily true.

Remember the four friends who brought a paralytic to Christ to be healed? They could not reach Jesus because of the crowd, so they opened a hole in the roof of the house Jesus was in and let the man and his bed down. The Bible records that when Jesus saw the faith of the man's friends, He forgave the man's sins and healed him (Mark 2:5–12). The patient was healed, yet he was not the one whose faith Jesus commended. It wasn't the patient's faith that Jesus acted on, but that of his friends.

Jesus was very impressed with the faith of the centurion who asked Jesus to heal his servant, who was at the centurion's home. Jesus immediately wanted to go to the servant, but the centurion told him that wasn't necessary, that Jesus just needed to say the word and it would be done (Matt.

8:5–10). The centurion's faith got Jesus' attention.

Still, faith *was* the motivating factor in all these healings. But what about the healing of Lazarus (that is, if you want to call raising someone from the dead a healing, and I do!)? His sisters, Mary and Martha, didn't have faith; his believing friends didn't have faith. Lazarus certainly didn't have faith (he was dead! Yet Jesus raised him from the grave (John 11:1–45). Where was the faith?

Yes, faith has great power. If only we had faith the size of a mustard seed, we could move mountains, right? *That is, if moving that mountain is in God's plan.*

We expect God to stick to His healing promises, don't we? After all, He's God. He can't go back on His Word. He chose to give us those promises, so we can rightfully claim them. In fact, we do more than claim them—we demand them! But is that right?

An evangelist and dear friend of mine once told me that he demanded his rights from his wife, and sure enough, she replied not only with rights, but also with some powerful lefts!

Of all of God's attributes, the one we tend to forget the most is that He is sovereign. He has supreme authority, and He is in control.

> And God said unto Moses, I AM THAT I AM: and he said; Thus shalt thou say unto the children of Israel, I AM hath sent me unto you.
>
> —EXODUS 3:14

> The LORD killeth, and maketh alive: he bringeth down to the grave, and bringeth up. The LORD maketh poor, and maketh rich: he bringeth low, and lifteth up.
>
> —1 SAMUEL 2:6–7

God is all powerful. He is over all things—even the desperate situations in our lives. It is my humble opinion that it is not our position to demand anything from God, but to rest assured that He will always do what is best for us, no matter how bizarre our circumstances.

Yet God appeals to us to call on Him when we have needs. And prayer is the natural language of the godly and the ungodly in desperate moments. When cancer gives people a due date to turn in their bodies, even the most devout atheists will explore the possibility of someone more powerful—someone who can come to their rescue. Desperate times become times to pray. And as we have learned, prayer has power.

THE INFLUENCE OF PRAYER

AS WE ALREADY noted in chapter eight, cardiologist Randolph Byrd put prayer on the scientific map with his study in the coronary unit of the San Francisco General Hospital. Even committed opponents like Dr. William Nolan, a noted author who has spoken out against faith healing, acknowledged that "this study will stand up to scrutiny.... Maybe we doctors ought to be writing on our order sheets, 'Pray three times a day.' If it works, it works."[1]

Dr. Larry Dossey, in his best-selling book *Healing Words,* says, "If the technique studied [by Dr. Byrd] had been a new drug or a surgical procedure instead of prayer, it would almost certainly have been heralded as some sort of breakthrough."[2]

To date, some 350 research papers have been published in scientific journals about the power of prayer. Interestingly enough, about half "prove" that it works, and the other half "prove" that it doesn't.

So, is God only 50 percent effective? Testing God's healing capabilities, if you want to look at it that way, has always struck me as irreverent, to say the least. But even in Dr. Byrd's study, "God's success rate" was not close to 50 percent. Some may say that the people praying were not "born again" or "Spirit filled." Be that as it may, no matter who prays, *the success rate is never 100 percent.*

It is as unreasonable to expect that God heals everybody as it is to expect that God answers everybody's prayers with a yes. When patients can accept this, they rise to a new level of peace.

Let's imagine for a moment that God "answered" every prayer for healing. What would happen? The world would probably be overpopulated by now. And think about how chaotic everything would be. Someone would be praying fervently for rain for his garden, while his next door neighbor would be praying for no rain because of an outside wedding that day. Each is asking God to be with him in his corner of a boxing match. What would happen? It would be impossible for God to be more than 50 percent effective, even if He wanted to.

LEVELS OF PRAYER

FINALLY, THERE IS prayer, and then there is *prayer.* After a national catastrophe President Clinton usually tells the affected people that his prayers are with them. I'm sure that none of us picture him on his knees, praying fervently for the people. But if Billy Graham says he is praying for the suffering, we do picture him kneeling before God, interceding for them.

So there are different types and levels of prayer.

The intrinsic power of any prayer

There is "magic" in prayer. In spite of many Christian beliefs, any prayer has power. In other words, the *source* of some power lies in prayer itself.

According to William G. Braud of the Mind Science Foundation, these methods are duplicable, regardless of religious beliefs or disbelief, if you follow the protocol.[3]

Different techniques of prayer are used effectively by

many health and spiritual practitioners around the world. The word *prayer* is used indiscriminately for meditation, relaxation, biofeedback, visualization, intentionality, imagery—techniques all used by both health professionals and mystics over generations. Some of the experts have developed skills so that they can control the growth of plants and even bacteria using these techniques. Others are so careful with their power that they refuse to use it for any type of destructive effort, even destruction of deadly viruses.

Most of us have experienced to some extent the power of our minds by staring at someone and making them turn to look at us, for instance. By God's design, the power of the mind is amazing and can promote healing or sorrow. In many cases, patients deposit such faith in their doctors that they will respond directly to the doctor's confidence in the treatment. If the physician conveys a sense of failure, the patient will not respond well, but if the doctor shows excitement and belief in the program, the patient recuperates faster.

We all have heard patients say that as soon as they consulted their beloved doctor, they got better even before taking the first pill. That is the reason for double-blind studies in which neither doctors nor patients know which patient is taking the placebo and which is taking the drug. If the doctor knew, the doctor's attitude could sway the results if he believed the therapy was effective.

By the same token, positive, happy, cheerful patients in general do better and improve faster than the pessimists because the power of the mind is effective to construct or to destroy. This complies with the natural laws of creation. The power of the mind is there for all to use. You may want to consider thanking the Creator for this ingenious trait.

The supernatural power of God's intervention
The intrinsic power of any prayer, along with the power of

the mind, is somewhat easy for people, including scientists, to accept. However, the supernatural power of prayer—that is, the intervention into our lives by God—is very controversial.

In this model, the act of prayer has no intrinsic capabilities, no "magic." Any power and glory revealed comes only from above, from God. Miracles from this kind of prayer are discriminate and supernatural. They are without rational explanation or pattern. They may happen to Christians, Buddhists or agnostics. Healing may occur after fervent prayer or no prayer at all.

At Oasis of Hope Hospital, we maintain a constant prayer chain for all our patients. When a child with cancer is in our hospital, my staff suffers more emotionally than they do with other patients. Even other patients start saying things like, "I would rather God take me than that child." Then when a child dies, we are perplexed. We prayed over the child, anointed the child with oil and were all in agreement for the healing, but the child never recovered. Why?

Some may be critical of a God who seems so unpredictable, who often makes no sense. The only explanation I have is that we see only in part while God sees the whole. He has a master plan, and what must come to pass will come to pass.

Our finite minds are incapable of grasping God, and I believe this is by design. If we were able to understand God and His ways, we would rely on that understanding. An easy formula would lead to the manipulation of God's power to meet our capricious needs. Then, instead of depending on God, we would depend on our own ability to master the formula.

God does not want that. He wants us to be utterly dependent on Him. Some agnostics criticize God because they think He is manipulating us like puppets. (Try puppeteering your sixteen-year-old!) Conversely, God would be the puppet if He acquiesced to our every wish or answered our every prayer with a yes. Now that's an ugly thought.

The Bible teaches us to "trust in the LORD with all your heart and lean not on your own understanding; in all your ways acknowledge him, and he will make your paths straight" (Prov. 3:5, NIV). When Jesus was asked by the disciples why He spoke in parables, He replied, "So that they will not understand." (See Mark 4:12.) So we are told to trust, and we can expect that we won't understand everything. And that's OK.

For ages, theologians and philosophers have tried to figure out God, something I believe to be a futile endeavor. In my opinion, God's attitude and actions let us know, in no uncertain terms, just who is in charge. They demonstrate His authority and sovereignty. We may reject His sovereignty, an action that leads to desperation, or embrace it and receive consolation.

The advantage Christians have is eternal. Some people may pray for healing and be healed. We can pray for healing, and if we are healed—great! If not, we still have eternal life with Christ.

THE BIG PICTURE

FROM OUR FINITE perspective we have difficulty grasping the concept that God is in charge even if we don't understand how it all is working out. But if we place ourselves outside the limits of time, if we see from eternity's perspective, we realize that our lives occupy only a fraction of the timeline. God answers prayer from this perspective, according to a master plan that is in tune with and beneficial for all of creation in an eternal consensus.

If we accept this perspective, it becomes obvious that all prayers *are* answered, that God is always 100 percent effective. From the human perspective, however, if God does not comply with our wishes, then that prayer is written off as a failure or as unanswered. But sometimes no *is* the answer, because it complies with the eternal perspective for the good of all. When we accept that, then the context of Paul's exhortation becomes clearer: "And we know that all things work together for good to them that love God, to them who are the called according to his purpose" (Rom. 8:28).

The Book of Job is a must-read for everyone. Job was without sin when calamity struck. This righteous man was worthy of having his love for and dedication to God tested to the extreme. He was wealthy with a wonderfully blessed family. But in one day he lost his family and all his possessions. When Job questioned God strongly on why those adversities were happening to him, God answered by sharing a glimpse of the "big picture" with him.

That view helped Job take into account who God really was as well as the minuscule part his own life and circumstances played in the vastness of God. Job was totally humbled. He realized that humans do not have the God-given right to ask why or understand everything that occurs. We are to trust and believe instead. When Job was able to surrender all doubt and questioning to the Lord, the Lord blessed Job two times over.

ABANDONED TO GOD

THE LORD'S PRAYER and the prayer Jesus prayed on His last night on earth are the two most powerful teachings on prayer with eternal perspective. When Jesus taught us how to pray, He said, "Thy kingdom come. Thy will be done" (Matt. 6:10). Then again, when He prayed alone on the Mount of Olives moments before Judas would betray Him, He said, "Father, if you are willing, take this cup from me; yet not my will, but yours be done" (Luke 22:42, NIV).

Once I asked a patient of mine who experienced what we call "spontaneous remission" (the unexplained disappearance of cancer) if he had fasted and prayed. Almost with shame he confided in me that he actually had done nothing.

His trust in God was such that he accepted the diagnosis of cancer as God's will. And his tumor disappeared. Whether we believe or not, God's will *will be done.*

Dr. Yujiro Ikemi of Kyushu University in Fukuoka, Japan, reported five cases of spontaneous remissions in 1975. The common denominator in these fantastic cures was the fact that the patients surrendered to their diagnosis of terminal cancer with an attitude of gratitude and acceptance that this was best for them. They all were members of the Shinto religious sect, but still the message was, "Your will, not mine." This is a tremendous example of the power of submission to the master plan.

There is true freedom in submission. When we are finally able to abandon ourselves completely to God and trust that His will is the best thing that can possibly happen to us, we experience true liberty. Jesus prayed for what He desired, but He understood that God's everlasting plan would ultimately be best. He prayed for life, but instead He went through pain, humiliation, agony and even death. Now we understand that God's master plan required temporary suffering in order to provide salvation to all.

I urge you to pray for healing and for the desires of your heart, as the Bible says. But be quick to recognize the wisdom and sovereignty of God's eternal perspective.

THE ISSUE IS LIFE

PERHAPS YOU'VE HEARD that just two things in life are certain: death and taxes. That is true, but the real question is, Are they so terrible? Taxes provide us good services. Americans complain about them, but if they lived in countries where people do not have these services, they would appreciate paying taxes to get them.

And then there's death. "Death," says Dr. Patch Adams, "is not a failure, but the last act of life."[4]

201

Since death is inevitable, it is really not the issue here. Life, not death, should be our focus. Life is to be enjoyed and cherished. Evolutionists, creationists and everyone else agrees that life is a gift. The point is not that we die, but how we have lived.

So let's discover how to really live—whatever amount of life we have.

13

Restoring the Power of Hope

MANNY RODRIGUEZ, A wealthy yuppie of thirty-five, came to see me because of advanced cancer of the stomach. As I pondered his poor prognosis, I started to preach to him positivism and the uplifting of the spirit.

"You don't understand, doctor," he interrupted. "Cancer has been the best thing that ever happened to me. I've been very successful in business, but that consumed me. I did not have time to appreciate all the blessings, the truly meaningful blessings that God has given me. Now that I have cancer, every minute of the day is precious to love my abandoned beautiful wife, to play and cradle my children, to absorb a sunset. Life is awesome, and I will enjoy it to the fullest."

I believe with all my heart that cancer can be managed much better if patients can trust God and enjoy their days to the fullest. Let's see what the first steps are.

MIND OVER MALIGNANT MATTER

Fear is faith in the negative.

Cancer is much more than a physical threat. The fear

factor cancer generates is off the scale. I frequently hear people say with conviction, "I'd rather die of a heart attack than get cancer." Many people would even go so far as to say, "I'd rather die than get cancer." Death is much less feared than cancer. Therein lies one of the fueling factors of cancer: fear.

We have already discovered that stress causes our immune systems to become depressed, so they can't fight off sickness as well. Fear immediately throws the body into the stress mode, commonly referred to as "fight or flight." The body then produces hormones to give it a sudden boost of energy and strength to overcome an immediate threat. This is a lifesaver if you need to get away from a shark, but you can never escape the threat of cancer. So, if the body is constantly stressed by this fear, the production of hormones can become excessive.

One of the hormones produced is cortisol, which depresses the production of T cells and NK cells (natural killer cells). The T and NK cells are the mighty warrior cells God put in our immune system to protect us from all the adversaries to our health, from the common cold to cancer, from the simple to the complex. So, fear physiologically depresses those cells, thereby promoting the potential for cancer.

If you do not have cancer, the fear of it increases the probability of a future diagnosis. If you have cancer, your fear will increase the devastation caused by cancer. Why? Fear is a natural ally of cancer. It does an "inside job" by depressing our immune system.

Fear—another god

Jesus taught that we should not be anxious or fearful. But with so many threats to our health like cancer, drive-by shootings and car accidents, how can we avoid being fearful? The answer is by the fear of the Lord.

When you fear God, you know Him and understand that He has the power and desire to protect you. Any fear other than the fear of God can be categorized as the fear of man and the doubt of God. To take it to an extreme point, the fear of anything or anyone other than God is idolatry. Why?

If you fear something greatly, you are experiencing a lapse of memory that God can and will make sure that only the best things for your life will come to pass. If you lack trust that God is in control, then you will fear other things. Whatever you fear the most, in essence, is your god.

I encourage you to focus on God and not fear cancer. You wouldn't want to fear cancer to the point of making it your god, would you? Don't bow down to cancer. Stand up to it, and let it know that the Lord your God will give you victory over cancer.

The self-fulfilling prophecy

Self-fulfilling prophecy is a term used in psychological circles to describe how what is said about people or what they say about themselves comes to pass. The scientific studies of immune-depressing factors help to explain the physical mechanism of this.

In the Bible it is written, "As [a man] thinketh in his heart, so he is" (Prov. 23:7). If you think you are going to die because you have cancer, you're increasing your chances. Your immune system will lay down its armor to honor you. It will not humiliate you by proving your morbid belief wrong.

Fear is a function of negative faith—belief that the negative thing can or will happen. If you fear cancer, then you have faith (a negative faith) that you will get it or will die from it. Faith is a powerful part of the self-fulfilling prophecy.

When the woman with the issue of blood touched the hem of Jesus' garment, she was healed. Jesus said to her, "Your faith has made you well" (Mark 5:34, NKJV). She believed and told herself that if she could touch even the hem of Jesus' garment, she would be well. And so she was. Her body fulfilled the prophecy she gave it.

Since you're going to believe something, believe the positive instead of the negative. Positive faith is so powerful. Dr. Bernie Siegel encourages his patients who opt for radiation and chemotherapy to visualize the treatments working against the cancer and not producing the negative side effects. They draw pictures of the positive work the therapy is doing. Dr. Siegel has documented how their positive attitudes toward cancer and their treatment choice truly generate better outcomes than the outcomes other cancer patients have.[1]

An attitude of hope

Other profound truths about the power of attitude were uncovered by Viktor Frankl, a prisoner in Auschwitz during the Holocaust. He explains in his book *Man's Search for Meaning* how the prisoners were so intimately acquainted with death that they could accurately predict the time a person would die, sometimes with a margin of error as little as a few minutes.

Oddly enough, a key indicator that a person was going to die within a few days was that he would start smoking his cigarettes. You see, in the prison camps cigarettes were used as money. People didn't smoke them, just as you would not light up a $20 bill. If a person started smoking his cigarettes, it meant one thing—he had given up hope.

Frankl wrote about the direct correlation between the absence of hope and death. If you believe there is no hope, then there isn't hope for you. This negative faith will fulfill a negative prophecy.

Your attitude toward cancer is vital. The secret to preventing or curing cancer begins in your mind and your heart. Fear and negative faith work against you. I believe it is critical for people to have the proper mental attitude in order for healing to take place.

A number of spiritual counselors work with my patients toward the specific objective of empowering them with the emotional and spiritual attitudes to overcome cancer. We help people to shift from their fear of cancer to their faith in God and themselves to conquer cancer. These new positive beliefs, in fact, stimulate the immune system and put their God-ordained defense mechanism back on duty.

When Dee Simmons found out she had cancer of the breast, she underwent a successful modified radical mastectomy and went in remission. However, her oncologists wanted to do more "preventative" therapy because, at age forty-five, there was a high risk for recurrence of this very aggressive malignancy.

Since her active life did not allow for the side effects of this aggressive prevention method, she decided to look into alternatives. So she traveled all over the world in her private jet to research every option that existed. Finally, she found Oasis of Hope Hospital.

As a Christian she believed that God had already provided, through the doctors, a miracle. But she didn't rest on her laurels; she knew she would have to work at staying well. After her research tour and a three-week stay in our hospital, she came to understand that the cancer had appeared because her immune system had failed. Thus, she made it her goal to put her defenses back together and get them in better shape than ever. This was the only way to keep any recurrence of this tumor from attacking her again.

As most patients who come to that conclusion discover, this is no simple task. The amount of supplements available are staggering, and patients interested in this avenue often end up taking hundreds of pills every day. New products appear on the market daily, it seems, and patients become confused as to what is best.

When Dee ran into this problem, she hired some of the best chemists to put together a formula that would incorporate all her needs into one product. This concoction was quite easy to take, and it made her life functional again.

Dee is remarkable in that, even though she has been an inspiration to many because of her testimony of victory over cancer, she didn't stop there. After experiencing what God had done for her, she began a crusade to fight cancer by giving cancer victims hope and resources. Soon, more and more of her fellow patients wanted to take her concoction for the immune system, so she decided to make it available commercially. Believe me, she does not need this kind of trouble, but she does want to share what God has done for her.

I tell my patients that when God gives them a miracle, they have the responsibility to maintain that miracle. So it cannot be business as usual. The lifestyle that led them to disease, if not changed, will bring the disease back. If that happens, people often blame God for not doing it right the first time. Oops!

Perhaps you think that it is easy to live life victoriously when your cancer is gone. Well, some people are thrilled with their new lease on life, but they go back to doing everything the same as before cancer struck. I'm not referring just to eating habits, but also to the same defeated attitudes, the same absence of living life to the fullest.

Not so with Dee Simmons. Not only has she been a good steward of her miracle, she has also helped others prevent and fight cancer. She took something that could have been devastating and fearful and turned it into a new way to live her life with vitality and meaning. Now that is victory! (If you haven't read Dee's personal story yet, it is in Appendix E.)

Sometimes cancer inspires people to be victors, and

sometimes it leaves them victims. And in my opinion, it's a matter of choice, not diagnosis.

When Susie arrived at our hospital, everyone leapt into action. The condition of this fragile nine-year-old was desperate. She was lethargic but conscious, in spite of her striking paleness. The nurses prepared medications and IVs. Her bed was surrounded with the commotion of people attending to her and requesting all kinds of supplies.

Susie's father was on the edge of a nervous breakdown. Because of various chemotherapy protocols, his daughter's cancer had been in and out of remission for two years. But this last time she just didn't respond to therapy, and the girl had been sent home to die.

While we were attending to his daughter, he went to the next room to pray. We could clearly hear his cry for God's mercy in spite of the buzz we were making in trying to save his daughter's life.

Susie's father was no stranger to prayer. As one of the lay elders in a modern church, he had seen miracles take place after prayer. In fact, several members of the church he attended agreed with his feeling that God would heal his daughter.

After pertinent medical intervention, fluids and blood transfusions, we were able to stabilize Susie's condition. She finally went to sleep with a restful face. Her father's desperation, however, did not diminish one bit.

Our intervention stabilized the girl, but Susie's dad knew that the improvement was only temporary. The disease was still as deadly as it had been a few hours previous. During the next two days, nobody saw him leave his daughter's side. He was there constantly, praying and reminding God of all the promises in the Bible.

The child had not uttered a word in all those hours of distress. I still remember with a broken heart her face as she looked at me with gratitude and a faint smile. Her only means of communication during our brief moments together was holding my hand very tightly.

When she died, there arose a upheaval that none of us had ever experienced before—and believe me, in a cancer care unit, we often see desperation and defeat along with crying and rebellion. But Susie's father was in such pain and disbelief that he could not hold himself in. He just could not accept God's mistake. How could God do this to him, a man who had served Him and told others about His mercies and goodness all the time? It was not fair; it was just not right.

This man prayed with anger and conviction for his daughter to resuscitate. But of course, she didn't. Susie rested in peace, but her father had fallen victim to the stronghold of cancer. Yet, as the father of five children, my heart connected with this man's cry for answers.

I pray for him even today, for his reconciliation with the God who didn't meet his expectations. I pray that his experience with cancer does not hold him a victim and destroy his life. Cancer consumed his daughter's life, but my prayer is that it will not consume her father's soul.

I pray for all those whose lives are trapped as victims of this foul disease, because victory over cancer, even in this most treacherous of situations, is a real possibility.

Victory over cancer should not be defined as the eradication of the tumor. Victory over cancer is being able to enjoy life whether cancer exists or not, even if physical death may be a possibility. When you can put your mind over malignant matter, you will be able to go the distance, just as Jack Riley did.

People may wonder why I consider Jack Riley a success story even though he passed away. It's because Jack accomplished more from the time he was diagnosed with cancer until his death than most of us will in a lifetime. He converted the fear of cancer into fuel for his mission. You can find his story in Appendix F, but let me share a little of it with you.

In mid-life Jack Riley started running triathlons, those grueling races in which the participants swim, bike and run. As he got older, he continued racing, winning many awards. Then Jack received the diagnosis of prostate cancer. He underwent many conventional treatments, including two cryosurgeries and fifty-two radiation treatments. Through it all, Jack kept racing.

In fact, he ran two transnational, one-man triathlons, raising money for cancer research and visiting children's cancer centers at the same time. He always maintained a winning spirit, encouraging others with cancer to keep on going. The day after a radiation treatment, he ran the Los Angeles Marathon!

At age sixty-five, Jack learned that he had less than a year to live. He was never bitter or resentful. Instead, he lived each day to the fullest.

At our hospital, Jack received immune-system enhancement treatments, which helped to contain his cancer. But he was in constant pain as he ran his last transnational triathlon. A bone scan revealed that the aggressive cancer that previously attacked his prostate had spread to his lower back, hip, pelvic and spinal areas.

In the last phase of his life, Jack wasn't dwelling on dying; he was concentrating on living. He went the way that he wanted to—serving others and fighting for a cure to cancer. And along the way his unshakable spirit inspired millions. Though he died, he was truly a victor. Jack never complained or grumbled—he was too busy living life!

Spending my life in the midst of death and dying is draining. When my spirit is burdened and my shoulders sag, I remember Jack and so many others of my hero patients. Then a wave of warmth invades my whole being, and my eyes well up with tears. This spiritual force empowers me to keep on keeping on.

14

Victory—Yours to Seize!

THE HOPE OF living cancer free is the hope of victory over it. For some, victory lies in long-term prevention, something only to be enjoyed by future generations. For others, victory depends on finding the cure—without a cure, they are left hopeless. For me, *victory over cancer is a matter of choice.*

If you are cancer free because the disease has not stricken you, be thankful, but also be responsible. Do what you can to prevent it. Be a successful risk manager, adopt a personal and family policy of health—but above all, acknowledge that by grace you are enjoying the gift of health.

If you are cancer free through successful treatment, be thankful to your doctor and to the source of the doctor's healing power—God. If your cancer has miraculously vanished, don't thank the heavens, circumstances or fate. Thank God for His generous gift.

Yes, it is wonderful to be rid of cancer, no matter the categories into which you fall.

However, if you have recently been diagnosed with cancer, I pray that God will fill you with His grace and provide the miracle for which you are waiting and praying. You may not believe in God; nevertheless, expect a miracle. For whether you believe or not, God is a God of mercy. If you have won the battle against cancer, but it has come back, do not despair. As with most things in life, miracles come in pairs.

For those of you who are veteran cancer warriors, who feel tired of the uphill battle, who have had too many disappointments and who are certain that the hope of living cancer free is an illusion, let me challenge your desperation and pessimism. Come with me and explore an incredible avenue of new hope for you. "While there is life, there is hope." Let this old adage give you that little push you need to reach deep inside and seek victory.

WHAT IS VICTORY?

"I WILL BE conquered; I will not capitulate." That was one of the last statements of Samuel Johnson (1709–1784), the famous English author. Despite the tribulation you are facing, you can still choose whether you will be a victim or a victor. Let me define victory for you.

When the plane's door opened and the girls marched down the stairs, the crowd went crazy. By the people's cheering, you would have thought the team had won. The Chinese female national team came home to a hero's welcome after losing the final in the women's soccer world championship. As defending champions, second place was not so special. But the fans were bursting with sheer appreciation and support. Victory, in all practicality, is a matter of perception.

If you ask me who my heroes are, I will tell you that they are my patients who found meaning in the midst of suffering. That is victory.

It touches me so deeply when I see my patients selflessly praying for the healing of others with cancer. I have been greatly moved by their positive attitudes and inspired by their ability to give to others when their own needs are so great. Some of my patients accept prayer, but healing isn't their priority. Why not? Because they have found meaning, even in a cancer crisis.

I remember my nephew Daniel praying with our patients on Worldwide Cancer Prayer Day on June 5, 1998. He asked one patient if he would like us to pray for his healing. The patient's response was that healing would be a bonus, but it really wasn't necessary. When Daniel asked what he meant, out came a lovely story of his personal victory.

His wife of many years had been such a blessing, he told Daniel, that it far outweighed the health crisis he was experiencing. God had already "overblessed" him, and he needed nothing more.

He also confided that two of his three children had broken marriages. But when the diagnosis of his cancer came, his children started praying together, and the marriages were reunited as a result of their united prayer. A number of his friends came to know the Lord because they started praying for him. Wisely, he concluded that if it took him getting cancer to see all of that eternal healing take place, it was worth it for him. That was his victory.

Victory just moves the boundary lines of our lives; it can't abolish them forever. Even victory has its inherent problems. Granted, they are more agreeable than the problems of defeat, but they are no less difficult. It is indeed common that victors are by victories destroyed. On the other hand, we all have heard true stories of people whose defeat, paradoxically, became their path to greatness.

And then there is neutrality, an even score. When asked about who won in the Cuban missile crisis, Nikita Khrushchev answered, "They talk about who won and who lost. Human reason won. Mankind won." A very diplomatic account of not winning, but not losing.

For the new generation of athletes the purpose of competing is to win. Would it surprise you if I said that is a misguided goal? People used to play just for the sake of competing. The truth is, if we fight cancer to win, to eradicate it, we will most likely suffer disappointment. That goal is near-sighted. But if we fight cancer to be liberated from it, the results will more than likely be realized.

It should not be the eradication of cancer for which we take up arms. Instead, we can lay down our arms in order for One who is more powerful than us to fulfill a higher purpose. This requires understanding our limitations and relying on God's limitlessness.

A New Measure of Health

THE ART OF healing runs in my veins, not only because my father is a doctor—the best I know—but also because I have been close to suffering patients since I was young. I was nine years old when my father decided to treat cancer patients with alternative therapies.

Today, not even the most orthodox practitioner of medicine rejects the possible benefits that alternative therapies can bring to a patient. But in 1963, my father was ostracized for his unconventional attempts to alleviate the suffering of patients. No hospital wanted to provide the services he wanted for his patients; no colleague wanted to be seen close to him. He was isolated and exiled from the medical community.

When out-of-town patients needed hospitalization, he would bring them home. My sisters, brother and I would relinquish our rooms for those hurting, dying people. Their suffering burdened me, and I wanted to learn to heal them. Our whole family was involved in helping patients improve, in helping them cope.

This experience nurtured within me a constant passion

for healing, and it seeded the respect and appreciation I have for good health. At an early stage of my life, I became conscious that life is fragile and there is such a thing as physical immortality. The preservation of God's gift of health is, I'm convinced, a moral *duty*.

I enjoy life; I live every day with intensity as if it were my last. The majority of human beings behave as though death were no more than an unfounded rumor. I have spent—no, I have invested—time writing this book to entice you to live life and live it abundantly.

A healthy life can become so routine that we take it for granted. I encourage you to start measuring your health by a new standard. Gauge it by your affection for a breathtaking morning sunrise or the inaugural flower of spring. If the first snowfall and the beauty of the night sky do not mesmerize you, if the prospect of spending time with family and friends is a chore, then you need to be awakened to the joy of being alive.

Of all the antisocial activities there are, the worst is disinterest in health. Henrik Ibsen, a nineteenth-century Norwegian dramatist, said it best: "People who don't know how to keep themselves healthy ought to have the decency to get themselves buried, and not waste time about it." Life and health are free, and thus it takes a long time to begin to appreciate them.

The Harmony of Life and Death

LIFE ITSELF IS a paradox. Health and illness, beauty and ugliness, perfection and imperfection—all these coexist. Pleasure cannot exclude pain. Without contrasts and differences our existence would have little meaning. So health and its enemy, disease, shape a transitional momentum between life and death. We know that death will happen to all of us; we just don't want to be there when it happens.

217

But in the blink of an eye, health is lost—many times temporarily, sometimes permanently. How does one cope, much less enjoy life in this condition? Someone once wrote, "It is not death, but dying, which is terrible." Many of my patients feel a kinship with that statement. I have experienced, with many patients, the feeling of desperate impotence in the midst of pain. That is the time to pray for deliverance and the grace of a miracle.

Throughout my life my position on health has been unchanged. However, time and experience have brought about a metamorphosis in my relationship with death. For the longest time death was the enemy—my enemy. Death was to be defeated. Of course, crash courses in maturity teach everybody, even naíve doctors, that death is not the opposite of life. In fact, death is the vehicle that joins us with the majority.

I thought that striving for and reaching health was the expected—and only—goal. But life and death dance in perfect harmony in God's ways. Many judge God as cruel and insensitive to man's pain and agree with Shakespeare's famous phrase from *King Lear:* "As flies to wanton boys, are we to th' gods; they kill us for their sport." But no. Death gives room for life. Creation and destruction are a never-ending process.

Arrogant idealism strives to abolish death. If that happened, mankind would multiply itself millions upon millions, a horrible prospect. (To get a feeling for that, spend some time in Mexico City with its twenty-five million inhabitants). Elton John calls the cycle of life and death "The Circle of Life" in the beautiful score of the movie *The Lion King.* In essence, death could be considered a call of love if we accept it as one of the great eternal forms of life and transformation.

So I stopped my futile and pointless fight against death. I learned how important it is to love life, but also not to fear death. If I had read my Bible more carefully, I would have discovered that Jesus, not I, would be the one to conquer death: "The last enemy that shall be destroyed is death" (1 Cor. 15:26).

Meanwhile, death is with us, and if we cannot defeat it, our best bet is to join forces with it.

In a philosophical conversation about death and dying with Satoru Konishi, a good and profound friend, he recited a beautiful Native American poem to me, one whose author he could not remember. When he first heard the poem, it made such a deep impression on him that he learned it by heart, in spite of the fact that his English is quite limited. Here it is for you:

> Today is a very good day to die.
> Every living thing is in harmony with me.
> Every voice sings a chorus within me.
> All beauty has come to rest in my eyes.
> All bad thoughts have departed from me.
>
> Today is a very good day to die.
> My land is peaceful around me.
> My fields have been turned for the last time.
> My house is filled with laughter.
> My children have come home.
>
> Yes, today is a very good day to die.

Its message is so powerful and wise. Death should not surprise us; we should be prepared for it always. The spirit of the poem is accepting death with gratitude and without a sense of defeat. The disease that may be threatening the life of this poet is of no importance because it honors creation's design; he is looking forward to meeting the Creator. The poet is not begging for life to end; he is just transcending desperation.

The Hope of Living Cancer Free

THE ZONE OF PEACE

BEING AT PEACE with yourself is a wonderful experience, but when you are at peace with the One who made you, then you truly enter into "the zone"—that illusive place where every thing seems perfect. In the zone the points of reference are in places our minds cannot reach, but where our spirits are at home with and absorb the fullness of eternity.

"See in what peace a Christian can die." Joseph Addison, that inspiring English essayist, was in the zone when he uttered these dying words in 1719.

Jack Riley, our triathlete with cancer of the prostate, said that if God were going to heal him of cancer, he would ask instead for one more day with cancer so he could fight the fight for others less fortunate. That's being in the zone.

When you are blessed with a miraculous healing, you are a witness of God's grace. But the cure is not necessarily the physical disappearance of cancer. Total liberation from cancer is acknowledging that sickness, no matter how painful or grotesque, is only for a moment in the eternal scheme of God. Whether it goes away completely or comes back is secondary.

If you need to relate to someone who suffered as much as you and who experienced utter pain, listen to the apostle Paul:

> Whether we live, we live unto the Lord; and whether we die, we die unto the Lord; whether we live therefore, or die, we are the Lord's.
>
> —ROMANS 14:8

It was also Paul who said:

> Who shall separate us from the love of Christ? Shall tribulation, or distress, or persecution, or famine, or

220

nakedness, or peril, or sword? As it is written, For thy sake we are killed all the day long; we are accounted as sheep for the slaughter.

Nay, in all these things we are more than conquerors through him that loved us. For I am persuaded, that neither death, nor life, nor angels, nor principalities, nor powers, nor things present, nor things to come, nor height, nor depth, nor any other creature, shall be able to separate us from the love of God, which is in Christ Jesus our Lord.

—ROMANS 8:35–39, EMPHASIS ADDED

All these powerful, committed words have meaning only if we place ourselves in the same zone as Paul—the zone of the promised land. In that place of glory that is to come—heaven—there will be no more sorrow or pain.

If you are enjoying good health, or if God has miraculously healed you, that is *grace.* But we are able to cope with adversity because He provides the strength to withstand, with dignity and valor, the onslaught of cancer. In that place He shows us that the ultimate purpose for our suffering will be accomplished through His support and love, and that we are completely beyond the ravages of disease and death. And that, my friends, is amazing grace.

Indeed, today is a very good day to...live. Make today the day in which you choose to have the ultimate victory, because our hope of living cancer free is not utopian, but real, eternal and absolute.

Appendix A

**Estimated New Cancer Cases and Deaths
by Sex for All Sites, United States, 1999[1]**

Cancer Sites	Estimated New Cases			Estimated Deaths		
	Both Sexes	Male	Female	Both Sexes	Male	Female
All Sites	1,221,800	623,800	598,000	563,100	291,100	272,000
Oral cavity & pharynx	29,800	20,000	9,800	8,100	5,400	2,700
Tongue	6,600	4,300	2,300	1,800	1,200	600
Mouth	10,800	6,400	4,400	2,300	1,300	1,000
Pharynx	8,300	6,100	2,200	2,100	1,500	600
Other oral cavity	4,100	3,200	900	1,900	1,400	500
Digestive system	226,300	117,200	109,100	131,000	69,900	61,100
Esophagus	12,500	9,400	3,100	12,200	9,400	2,800
Stomach	21,900	13,700	8,200	13,500	7,900	5,600
Small intestine	4,800	2,500	2,300	1,200	600	600
Colon	94,700	43,000	51,700	47,900	23,000	24,900
Rectum	34,700	19,400	15,300	8,700	4,800	3,900
Anus, anal canal, & Anorectum	3,300	1,400	1,900	500	200	300
Liver & intrahepatic bile duct	14,500	9,600	4,900	13,600	8,400	5,200
Gallbladder & other biliary	7,200	3,000	4,200	3,600	1,300	2,300
Pancreas	28,600	14,000	14,600	28,600	13,900	14,700
Other digestive organs	4,100	1,200	2,900	1,200	400	800
Respiratory system	187,600	106,800	80,800	164,200	94,900	69,300
Larynx	10,600	8,600	2,000	4,200	3,300	900
Lung & bronchus	171,600	94,000	77,600	158,900	90,900	68,000
Other respiratory organs	5,400	4,200	1,200	1,100	700	400
Bones & joints	2,600	1,400	1,200	1,400	800	600
Soft tissue (including heart)	7,800	4,200	3,600	4,400	2,100	2,300
Skin (excluding basal & squamous)	54,000	33,400	20,600	9,200	5,800	3,400
Melanoma-skin	44,200	25,800	18,400	7,300	4,600	2,700
Other non-epithelial skin	9,800	7,600	2,200	1,900	1,200	700

Cancer Sites	Estimated New Cases			Estimated Deaths		
	Both Sexes	Male	Female	Both Sexes	Male	Female
Breast	176,300	1,300	175,000	43,700	400	43,300
Genital system	269,100	188,100	81,000	64,700	37,500	27,200
Uterine cervix	12,800		12,800	4,800		4,800
Vulva	3,300		3,300	900		900
Cancer Sites	Both Sexes	Male	Female	Both Sexes	Male	Female
Vagina & other genital, female	2,300		2,300	600		600
Prostate	179,300	179,300		37,000	37,000	
Testis	7,400	7,400		300	300	
Penis & other genital, male	1,400	1,400		200	200	
Urinary system	86,500	58,400	28,100	24,500	15,600	8,900
Urinary bladder	54,200	39,100	15,100	12,100	8,100	4,000
Kidney & renal pelvis	30,000	17,800	12,200	11,900	7,200	4,700
Ureter & other urinary organs	2,300	1,500	800	500	300	200
Eye & orbit	2,200	1,200	1,000	200	100	100
Brain & other nervous system	16,800	9,500	7,300	13,100	7,200	5,900
Endocrine system	19,800	5,400	14,400	2,000	900	1,100
Thyroid	18,100	4,600	13,500	1,200	500	700
Other endocrine	1,700	800	900	800	400	400
Non-Hodgkin's lymphoma	56,800	32,600	24,200	25,700	13,400	12,300
Multiple myeloma	13,700	7,300	6,400	11,400	5,800	5,600
Leukemia	30,200	16,800	13,400	22,100	12,400	9,700
Acute lymphocytic leukemia	3,100	1,800	1,300	1,400	800	600
Chronic lymphocytic leukemia	7,800	4,500	3,300	5,100	3,000	2,100
Acute myeloid leukemia	10,100	4,900	5,200	6,900	3,700	3,200
Chronic myeloid leukemia	4,500	2,700	1,800	2,300	1,300	1,000
Other leukemia	4,700	2,900	1,800	6,400	3,600	2,800
Other & unspecified primary	35,100	16,400	18,700	36,100	18,200	17,900

Excludes basal and squamous cell skin cancers and in situ carcinomas except urinary bladder. Carcinoma in situ of the breast accounts for about 39,900 new cases annually, and melanoma carcinoma in situ accounts for about 23,200 new cases annually. Estimates of new cases are based on incidence rates from the NCI SEER program 1979-1995. American Cancer Society, Surveillance Research, 1999.

Appendix B

Oasis of Hope Hospital

OASIS OF HOPE Hospital was founded in 1963 with the purpose of improving the physical, emotional and spiritual lives of its patients, staff and the worldwide community by providing a healing environment, patient-focused services and quality products. Dr. Ernesto Contreras, Sr., and his son Dr. Francisco Contreras have treated more than one hundred thousand patients, more than forty thousand of them Americans with cancer. Their focus is on the total well-being of their patients, not the eradication of disease. This has inspired them to develop quality doctor-patient relationships and offer therapies that uplift the body, mind and spirit.

Oasis of Hope offers natural, nontoxic and compassionate therapies and utilizes conventional cancer therapies when beneficial to the patient. No therapy that will compromise a patient's quality of life is administered by Oasis physicians. A heavy emphasize is placed on nutrition, detoxification and immune system stimulation—all with emotional and spiritual support. Patients and their companions are engaged in prayer, laughter and song as a normal part of the Contreras' treatment protocol.

The Hope of Living Cancer Free

Along with holistic cancer therapy programs, Oasis of Hope offers cancer and heart attack prevention programs as well as general hospital services. All of these programs are conducted in its modern 55,000-square-foot medical/surgical facility, which is located just three blocks off the Pacific Ocean, twenty miles south of San Diego, California, in Baja California, Mexico.

For more information about Oasis of Hope, call toll free from the United States at: 888-500-HOPE, or visit its Internet site at www.oasisofhope.com.

OASIS OF HOPE
P.O. Box 439045
San Ysidro, CA 92143
Toll-Free Telephone: 888-500-HOPE
Direct Telephone: (619) 690-8450
Fax: (619) 690-8410
Internet Site: www.oasisofhope.com
Email: health@oasisofhope.com

Related Internet Sites
www.kemsa.com
www.cancerresourcecenter.com
www.cancerprayerday.com
www.franciscocontreras.com

Appendix C

The Story of
Donald Factor

MY NAME IS Donald Factor. I was living in London in November 1986 when I was diagnosed with carcinoma of the lung that had spread to my liver. Basically the doctors in England didn't hold a lot of hope for me. They were very apologetic and offered a treatment that they thought might extend my life for a little while, but not for very long.

I didn't feel like accepting that prognosis, so I decided to go see Dr. Contreras. I'd met Dr. Contreras a few years before at a conference in England and was very impressed with his approach. He told us they used modern medicine combined with other natural things and a lot of love and faith. My wife and I moved from England to Los Angeles, and then we drove down to Tijuana to the hospital, where I was treated.

When I arrived, I was in an extremely weak condition. It was ten days after the original diagnosis, and the cancer had spread to my spine. I was in excruciating pain with my sciatic nerve affected, so I could hardly walk. I was losing weight rapidly, too.

They took a look at me at the Contreras clinic and were quite concerned. They too were not very optimistic about my future, but as Dr. Contreras, Sr., said, because both my wife and I were very committed to doing everything possible to beat the cancer, they were prepared to work with us.

To make a long story short, it succeeded. I knew Tijuana because I was born and raised in Los Angeles, and it was a place we used to go to do naughty things when we were teenagers. It wasn't ever a place that I associated with getting well, but rather a place that I associated with getting sick.

I was very impressed with the Contreras' clinic when I went inside and met the people. I had never experienced a hospital where the doctors would treat me as a human being instead of a bunch of symptoms or a disease walking through the door. Suddenly, there was a team of people there who were interested in me. They were involving me in the course my treatment would take. I was being asked, I was being informed and suddenly I was part of the team that was treating me. I wasn't just an object that was being treated, and that was tremendous. I realized there was another side of Tijuana that I never imagined possible in my youth.

This all happened in 1986. After the initial treatment and about a year of home therapy, I was totally clear of any sign of cancer. I went back regularly for check-ups, and after about three years of being in remission, the doctors said I was cured.

I said, "I thought in the cancer business you were never cured."

And they said, "Well, it is silly to keep writing down remission year after year. We'll see you whenever you want to come back." And that was it.

I already had a lot of ideas about the orthodoxy, I suppose I'd call it, of modern science. I was never happy with it. I had known people with HIV and AIDS, and I was always rather disturbed at the way that disease was treated. In those days it seemed that anyone who was diagnosed with HIV was dead within a couple of years. It didn't seem right to me.

It seemed to me that there was something else. I knew a bit about alternative and complementary medicine. My wife had been involved with some hands-on healing work before that, so I was very open to other ways of doing things. I had never had a direct experience myself as a patient being involved in a place where love and human kindness were actually applied as part of the program. I have to say it was a revelation.

My name has been given to people, and I have happily talked with them, telling them pretty much what I am telling you now. I think one of the main things that helped early on in my treatment was the use of a catheter, which was able to feed the medications directly into my liver. I think it was a Hickman catheter inserted into my umbilical vein that was able to stay in for about a year. It made taking all the medication much easier. One could simply inject whatever was needed into the end of a plastic tube, and it would get through the catheter to the body without the worry of needles and veins. That was wonderful. It made life much easier and the quality of the treatment better. It worked amazingly.

Appendix D

The Story of
Albert S.

I WAS DIAGNOSED WITH prostate cancer in 1986 at Los Angeles Community Hospital. I was in a treatment program with the hospital for about two years. At some point after the treatment, I was given about six weeks to live and was advised to get my personal affairs in order.

One of my four grandsons mentioned my grave illness to the members of his prayer group at work. They began to pray for me, and another prayer group member gave us a business card for the Hospital Ernesto Contreras, now Oasis of Hope Hospital. This individual had been successfully treated there himself.

We made an appointment with Dr. Lagos there, and I was hospitalized for two months for treatment. The treatment was successful, and in about six months I was examined and found to no longer have cancer.

In my visits to the hospital there, I have gained many friends over the years, including hospital staff and other patients. I am very grateful to Dr. Lagos and his kindness to me during my many trips to see him for treatment. He has been always very pleasant and professional in dealing with me. I am very grateful to the hospital staff for their care and concern for me over the years.

I thank God that I am a "survivor."

Appendix E

The Story of
Dee Simmons

TWELVE YEARS AGO I was diagnosed with breast cancer. I was devastated and shocked. First of all, I couldn't believe this could happen to me. I had never been sick, not even with a cold, and I had always considered myself to be a very healthy person. Immediately, I had a decision to make—*did I want to live, or did I want to die?* My choice was obvious.

Coming home from the hospital, I knew I must take charge of my life. I had just gone through an eight-hour modified radical mastectomy, and with my determination to survive, my journey began.

Fortunately, the first part of my journey took me to Oasis of Hope Hospital, then called Contreras Hospital, where I met and became a patient of Dr. Francisco Contreras. Immediately, my life was touched in a positive way with staff and environment that produced a reassurance of comfort, peace and healing. I was treated in not only a professional way, but as a family member.

The focus of Oasis was on the whole patient, not just the disease. With the assistance of Dr. Contreras and the hospital

233

staff, I learned how to take charge of my life, and this was the real journey, the journey of my healing. I soon became an avid student of nutrition and quickly learned how to apply the best of science and the best of nature to my personal life. I also learned health is the most valuable possession in life.

It's been said that the best things in life are free. Sometimes, however, those things that are most precious to us have a terrible cost. I consider our health to be one virtue that we hold most sacred. Unfortunately, some of us are stricken with a dreaded disease that threatens to cut short God's most special gift of life.

Cancer requires the ultimate battle. It forces a fight for life. Cancer is common and does not discriminate. Only a few years ago cancer was referred to as a condition too awful to talk about. Discussion, though often communicating knowledge, is a powerful weapon in the battle against cancer. Survivors know cancer can be conquered, and they speak a language of warfare. They truly have fought an enemy within—not simply the intruding cells, but their body's defenses, denial, anger and sometimes despair.

Many cancer survivors consider the disease to have been a gift in a horrible package, a message too dire to ignore: Life, which is indeed fleeting and precious, is a miracle and a gift from God.

I know hope is the most powerful medicine of all. Illness is an opportunity for growth, and the healing part comes from the ability to deal with whatever illness is troubling you. It's all about finding peace of mind.

How did an experience so tragic bring good into my life? It was a lesson to teach me where to turn to in a crisis. It pulled me into a dark valley, dropping me along the way—forcing me to rest and learn to trust Psalm 46:10: "Be still, and know that I am God."

He was in control. I emerged on the mountaintop, in the

same world but with a different appreciation of life and a closer relationship with my Savior. Yes, I touched the rose and felt the thorn. I've seen my life go from "vision to victory."

We cannot tell what may happen to us in the strange medley of life, but we can decide what happens within us...how we take it and what we do with it. That's what really counts in the end—how to take the raw stuff of life and make it a thing of worth and beauty. That is the test of living. The magic of life can never end, for it's filled with all life's greatest gifts—our family and friends.

If you are struggling with illness, remember the importance of a positive mental attitude, and do not give up hope. Arm yourself with knowledge about your illness, and become an active participant in your treatment plans. If you are well, please do not take your good health for granted.

In closing, I would like to reflect on someone who truly touched my life and taught me how to touch others. Dr. Francisco Contreras touches so many lives. I personally want to thank him once again for the unconditional commitment he made to me and continues to make to all his patients. My heart is full of gratitude to him and his staff. I salute each one for giving of themselves so that others are blessed with hope, strength and good health.

I will always remain grateful that Dr. Contreras and Oasis of Hope Hospital were a part of God's gift to me on my journey to victory over cancer. I thank Dr. Contreras for my treatment and direction of healing. With his help I've learned to speak and write words of encouragement and love to others who go through times of crisis and challenges. Today I am blessed to work closely with Dr. Contreras as I refer many people with a health crisis to Oasis of Hope...a place where people are committed to saving lives. One of the greatest blessings God can give to you is the gift of someone who cares. Dr. Contreras truly cares!

The Hope of Living Cancer Free

AUTHOR'S NOTE: I'm excited to announce that Dee's story has been published by Siloam Press in her book, *Ultimate Living!* This books tells her story and offers hope and encouragement to others who are experiencing crisis in their lives. Dee has been a fantastic model of what a person can do when faced with cancer. Now, she isn't just sitting on her miracle; she has a mission, vision and passion to help others overcome cancer, too.

Appendix F

The Story of Jack Riley

JACK RILEY WAS a senior triathlete. He entered races that involved three phases—swimming, biking and running. A grueling sport even for the young, Jack had begun running triathlons later in life.

A former drinker, smoker and junk-food advocate, Jack had traded in his bourbon glass for running shoes in mid-life. Jack competed in runs, marathons and triathlons 644 times. He had won more than 100 gold medals in his over-50 age division, and in 1985 at age 52 he made the *Guinness Book of World Records* by competing in 52 triathlons in one year.

After being diagnosed and treated for prostate cancer, Jack, a thirty-year resident of Alamo, California, became a community hero in 1996 when he was elected to carry the Olympic torch in San Francisco during the torch relay. He passed the flame on to the next runner, dipped his foot in the Pacific Ocean, then ran, biked and swam thirty-three hundred miles to the Olympic stadium in Atlanta, his personal Olympic torch in hand. He continued on until he arrived at the Atlantic Ocean.

The Hope of Living Cancer Free

In 1997 he ran, biked and swam seventeen hundred miles from Vancouver, Canada, to Tijuana, Mexico. Jack's runs took him through three hundred towns. Through the media, over fifteen million people were made aware of his quest. For Jack, the highlight of his trips was visiting children's cancer centers in the major cities and helping to cheer up the children and give them courage to fight their battle against cancer.

Through his runs Jack Riley personally raised over $130,000 for late-stage cancer research on prostate and breast cancer. His appearance on the steps of the state capitol building in Sacramento, California, after swimming the Sacramento River, helped motivate Governor Pete Wilson to sign a $27 million cancer support bill that he had just vetoed the year before.

Jack, who was not a doctor, scientist or researcher, had redesigned his life to be an important weapon he could use to win the ultimate battle and eradicate cancer from the earth. He told me, "If we can eradicate polio, there is no reason we can't eradicate cancer."

Jack had a tremendous capacity to look at the good side of life and live each day to the fullest. One day after the six-teenth of thirty-eight radiation treatments, Jack ran the Los Angeles Marathon and then flew home for his seventeenth treatment. The year before, after two hours of cryosurgery at a San Diego Hospital and three hours of rest, Jack danced an Irish jig with the nurse before he left the hospital. Three days after the operation he competed in a five-kilometer run.

Then, at age sixty-five, Jack learned that he had three to twelve months to live. The prostate cancer he had been diagnosed with five years earlier had spread. It was just a few weeks before the start of his third one-man trans-national triathlon. He was preparing for his most important race—the race against time.

The news was tough to swallow, but Jack was neither bitter nor resentful. He didn't pity himself or brood over his fate. In fact, he told people that God had blessed him to help lead the battle to eradicate cancer forever through his running of a 3000-mile triathlon that would raise money for cancer research.

Though he had just started a new series of radiation treatments when his triathlon began, he planned to leave the course a number of times to fly back to San Francisco for treatment, then return immediately to pick up the race where he left off.

In the last phase of his life, Jack wasn't dwelling on dying; he was concentrating on living. When I asked Jack Riley what his motivation was for attempting a physical feat that 99 percent of "healthy" people would be unable to do, he replied:

> I am a competitor. I guess it is just in my blood. If I can do this for a good cause, that's what life is all about. I will do this as long as I can, as long as God gives me the physical, mental and emotional ability. I see cancer as a competitor, and I don't dwell on my competition. I dwell on my own performance, which is in the hands of God.

One of Jack Riley's role models was Terry Fox, a twenty-year-old Canadian lad who lost part of his leg to cancer in 1980. Terry hobbled from the Atlantic Ocean toward the Pacific. He covered 3,321 miles before he was pulled off the course in Thunder Bay, Canada, because the cancer had metastasized into his lung. He died a few months later, but the Canadians raised twenty-four million dollars for cancer research as a result of his efforts.

Jack felt a close tie to Terry Fox though he had never met him. He enjoyed the fact that he was old enough to be Terry's grandfather, yet he was out there getting the job done. Though he had two legs and Terry only had one, Jack figured that he was equally challenged because his cancer had already metastasized and he had endured two cryosurgeries, fifty-two radiation treatments, energy-reducing hormones, a collapsed lung, an irregular heart beat and deep vein thrombosis (multiple blood clots) in both legs. Jack was excited that he completed two thousand more miles than Terry Fox did, but he never said he was better than Terry. He had an unshakable respect for Terry.

Jack Riley's dying wish was to raise enough funds for cancer research to finally eradicate the disease. So he set out on his third triathlon from the beach in Tijuana, Mexico, on the Worldwide Cancer Prayer Day—June 5, 1998. He planned to run, bike and swim the three thousand miles to the Statue of Liberty in New York City with his Olympic torch. He was wearing his well-worn "Cancer Doesn't Scare Me" T-shirt that had already survived five thousand miles of running, biking and swimming across the United States twice before.

A bone scan revealed that the aggressive cancer that previously attacked his prostate had spread to his lower back, hip, pelvic and spinal areas. He was in constant pain; he also had suffered a collapsed lung and had an irregular heartbeat. Jack received immune-system enhancement treatments at our Oasis of Hope Hospital in Tijuana, Mexico, which helped to contain his cancer.

On Jack Riley's third and final triathlon of hope, he made it from the Pacific Ocean through thirteen cities in California and Arizona. At New Mexico's border, his body gave out, though his spirit never did. Jack Riley passed away on July 1, 1998. His wife told me that he went the way that he wanted to—serving others and fighting for a cure to cancer.

Jack Riley was—and continues to be—a role model for

those with a cancer challenge; he kept a positive attitude through pain, radiation treatments, cryosurgeries, hormones, bone scans and resultant blood clots. "It is an understatement to say that he had a remarkable positive outlook. From the beginning, even during the most difficult treatments, he maintained his own very active lifestyle," said Dr. Michael Levine, a radiation oncologist at Mt. Diablo Medical Center in Concord, California.

"You don't run into people like Jack Riley. Most people adapt to the diagnosis and are as positive as they can be, but it's rare that people are this active," Levine added.

Another one of Jack Riley's doctors, Dr. Israel Barken, remarked, "The meaning of life to Jack was how he lived it day by day, and that is the lesson that other patients should learn from him." Jack took on death just as he had taken on life—passionately, aggressively and confidently.

Jack Riley's rich life had so many chapters to it. He had a personal relationship with Jesus Christ and a deep conviction that his life was in the hands of God. He worked with the American Heart Association, the American Cancer Society, cancer support groups and the Gold Medal foundation. Earlier he had worked for IBM and achieved excellence there.

Jack had even been in the military, where he picked up the call name "Eagle." The eagle, with its courage and independence, was a perfect symbol for Jack because he flew high and motivated others to reach for new heights, too.

In a day when it is difficult to find a hero, Jack Riley is one of mine because he had courage, commitment, love, integrity and focus. Jack Riley was a friend whose memory motivates me to do something meaningful with my life. When I feel challenged and even overwhelmed by the tasks of a day, I think of Jack. He had cancer, and yet he crossed the United States more than two times on his own power. What could I do if I made a real commitment? What can you achieve if you make an all-out effort?

Over the eight years that Jack Riley fought cancer, he came up with one hundred ways his disease benefited him. Some of them are written here in Jack's own words:

More courage
Count my blessings every day
A new sense of urgency
Spend more time with loved ones
Other problems seem smaller
Listen more to my feelings
More open to try new things
Better relationship with spouse
Feel more spiritual—I have turned it over to God
Tend to resolve outstanding issues in life
Feel free to be myself
Have more purpose in life
Try to be kinder, better person
An excitement about the challenge
Allow myself to think about the good times
Re-connect with old friends
Love and touch my pets more
Am less rigid
Opportunity to build faith, love and hope
Opportunity to build new friendships
Opportunity to relive great memories
Eat the right foods
Feel part of a "greater family" and mission
Love children more
Everyday events are more special
More prayers come my way
Am a better supporter
Meditate more
Listen to soothing music
Integrate positive thinking more

Appendix F

More consistent exerciser
Use relaxation techniques
Able to take a day off without guilt
Plan and do what I always wanted to do
Take soothing hot baths
Take advantage of massage
Pray more
Seek holy places
Allow more forgiveness
Am more compassionate
Use more positive affirmations
Use more positive visualizations
Have another level of awareness
Put more quality and balance in my life
My life feels more enriched
I am a better partner
Family get-togethers are more meaningful
My message is brighter
Spend less time on things that don't count
Less fear
Learning to celebrate whether I receive good news or
    bad news
Kiss my wife 1000 times more per year—I cherish her
    more
Value my wife and family more
Helped me to find the inner depths of my heart
Reaching out to distant members of my family
Everything has more meaning
I have an opportunity to correct some of my mistakes
If I have some self-doubts about doing something very
    bold and daring, they disappear very quickly
A deeper understanding of the greatness of the USA,
    Canada and Mexico
Design my life around what I love to do
I use the "love" word a lot more often

Notes

Introduction

1. American Cancer Society, *Cancer Facts and Figures* (Atlanta: American Cancer Society, 1999).
2. Ibid.

Chapter 1
Is There Hope for Living Cancer Free?

1. Ibid., 9, 15.
2. Ibid., 1.
3. Ibid.

Chapter 2
Breakthrough Strategies

1. This is a conclusion the author draws from the top ten causes of death in the United States (see www.health-status.com/top10.htm). The top ten total is 87.7 percent of all deaths. If you subtract the 1.8 percent of motor vehicle accidents and all other accidents, you will obtain 80.8 percent. Please note that the thesis that 80 percent of deaths is related to lifestyle is from the author.
2. Garduno Roberto, "Debajo de los niveles mínimos de nutrición, 24 millones," *La Jornada* (19 June 1994): 21.
3. Stephen Schoenthaler et. al., "The impact of a low food additive and sucrose diet on academic performance in 803 New York City Public Schools," *International Journal of Biological Research* 8, no. 2 (1986): 185–195.
4. Stephen Schoenthaler, "Institutional Nutritional Policies and Criminal Behavior," *Nutrition Today* 20, no. 3 (1986): 16.

5. Stephen Schoenthaler, "Diet and crime: An empirical examination of the value of nutrition in the treatment of incarcerated juvenile offenders," *International Journal of Biosocial Research* 4, no. 1 (1983): 25–39.
6. Anonymous, "The chemo's Berlin wall crumbles," *Cancer Chronicles* (December 1990): 4.

CHAPTER 3
EMPOWERED THINKING

1. John W. Yarbro. "Changing cancer care in the 1990s and the cost," *Cancer* 67 (1991):1718–1727. Note this last sentence is not an idea of Yarbro; he only says a "European view."
2. Source obtained from American Cancer Society Internet source: www.cancer.org/cancerinfo/basicfacts.
3. Arnold S. Relman, "The economic future of health care," *New England Journal of Medicine* 338, no. 25 (18 June 1998): 1855–1856.
4. Daniel Callahan, *False Hopes: Why America's Quest for Perfect Health Is a Recipe for Failure* (New York: Simon and Schuster, 1998).
5. Ibid.
6. Patrick Susskind, *The Perfume,* translated from Spanish into English by William H. Conrad (New York: Alfred A. Knoff, 1986).
7. Eustace Mullins, *Murder by Injection* (Virginia: The National Council for Medical Research, 1992), 137.
8. Michael Lemonick. "The killers. New viruses and drug-resistant bacteria are reversing human victories over infectious disease," *Time* (12 September 1994): 62–69.
9. Mullins, *Murder by Injection,* 8
10. Ibid.
11. Joseph D. Beasley, *The Betrayal of Health* (New York: Random House, 1991), 212.
12. George H. Malkmus, *Why Christians Get Sick* (Shippensburg, PA: Treasure House, 1997), 109.

Notes

CHAPTER 4
HOPE FOR A CURE

1. Mullins, *Murder by Injection,* 101.
2. Tim Beardsley, "A war not won," *Scientific American* (January 1994): 130–138.
3. Mullins, *Murder by Injection,* 101.
4. Beardsley, "A war not won," 130–138.
5. John C. Bailar III and Elaine M. Smith, "Progress Against Cancer?" *New England Journal of Medicine* 314, no. 19 (8 May 1986): 1231.
6. Ibid., 1226.
7. Ibid., 1231.
8. Source obtained from Internet: www.nci.gov/public/factbk96/hl.htm.
9. American Cancer Society, "Age-Adjusted Death Rates, 1930-1995," *Cancer Facts and Figures* (Atlanta: American Cancer Society, 1999).
10. Ibid.
11. Kedar N. Prasad, *Vitamins in Cancer Prevention and Treatment* (Rochester, VT: Healing Arts Press, 1994).
12. American Cancer Society, *Cancer Facts and Figures,* 9.
13. Karl A. Drlica, *Double-Edged Sword* (New York: Addisson-Wesley Publishing Company, 1994), 70–71.
14. John C. Bailar III and Elaine M. Smith, "Progress Against Cancer?" *New England Journal of Medicine* 314, no. 19 (8 May 1986): 1226–1232.
15. Ibid.
16. Ibid.
17. Anonymous, "The Chemo's Berlin Wall Crumbles," *Cancer Chronicles* (December 1990): 4.
18. Internet: www3.cancer.org/cancerinfo/basicfacts.
19. Ibid.
20. Thomas Balkany, "Why unconventional medicine?" *New England Journal of Medicine* 328, no. 4 (28 January 1993): 282.

CHAPTER 5
RESTORING THE INNER MAN

1. O. Carl Simonton, Stephanie Matthews-Simonton and James L. Creighton, *Getting Well Again* (New York: Bantam Books, 1992), 47–48.
2. This quotation comes from Bernie Siegel, *Love, Medicine and Miracles* (New York: Harper & Row, 1986), 80.
3. Simonton, *Getting Well Again*, 46.
4. Ibid., 52–53.
5. Siegel, *Love, Medicine and Miracles*, 82.
6. Madeleine Nash, "Stopping cancer in its tracks," *Time* (25 April 1994): 54–61.
7. Siegel, *Love, Medicine and Miracles*, 182(183.
8. Ibid., 183.
9. Ibid.
10. Ibid.
11. Ibid.

CHAPTER 6
RESTORING THE BODY

1. Beasley, *The Betrayal of Health*, 127.
2. Ibid., 115.
3. Internet source: Richard Boren, "The defeat of the dump in Sierra Blanca proves that if we all work together we can win," www.alphacdc.com/ien/blanca_2.html.
4. Comision Nacional de Derechos Humanos. Contaminación Atmosferica en México, sus causas y efectos (Mexico, 1992).
5. Beasley, *The Betrayal of Health*, 119.
6. Ibid.
7. David Susuki and Peter Knudtson, *Genetica* (Madrid: Editorial Tecnos, 1991).
8. Ibid.
9. Ibid.
10. Ibid.

Notes

11. Ibid.
12. Internet source: raleigh.dis.anl.gov/new/findingaids/epidemiologic/ hanford/intro.html.
13. Kristin Leutwyler, "Deciphering the breast cancer gene," *Scientific American* (December 1994): 18–19.
14. Internet source: Richard Boren, "The defeat of the dump in Sierra Blanca proves that if we all work together we can win," www.alphacdc.com/ien.blanca_2.html.
15. Beasley, *The Betrayal of Health,* 122–123.
16. Source obtained from the Internet: www.ocaw.org/txts/doc999902.htm.
17. Beasley, *The Betrayal of Health,* 125.
18. Ibid., 103.
19. Robert M. Kradjan, "Milk, The natural thing?" *Newlife* (November–December 1994).
20. Ibid.
21. Ibid.
22. Lauren Neegard, "FDA plans curbs on animal antibiotics," January 26, 1999, Associated Press.
23. Ralph W. Moss, Ph.D., "Cancer Risks Lurk in Hot Dogs and Burgers," *Cancer Chronicles* (July 1994).
24. Susan Preston-Martin et. al., "Maternal Consumption of Cured Meats and Vitamins in Relation to Pediatric Brain Tumors," *Cancer Epidemiology, Biomarkers and Prevention* 5, 599–605.
25. Internet source: "Mock Estrogen Tied to Cancer," www.abcnews.go.com/sections/living/DailyNews/estrogen0 311.html.
26. Ibid.
27. L.A. Brinton, "Ways that women may possible reduce their risk of breast cancer," *Journal of the National Cancer Institute* (1994).
28. Beasley, *The Betrayal of Health,* 104.
29. Ibid.
30. Ibid., 85.
31. Ibid., 87.
32. Ibid.

33. Ibid.
34. Deborah Schrag et al. "Decision analysis—Effect of prophylactic mastectomy and oophorectomy on life expectancy among women with BRCA1 or BCRA2 mutations," *New England Journal of Medicine* 336, no. 20 (15 May 1997): 1465.
35. Ibid.
36. Ibid.
37. Jennifer L. Kelsey and Leslie Bernstein, "Epidemiology and Prevention of breast cancer," *Annual Review of Public Health* 17 (1996): 53.
38. Ibid.
39. "The Cancer Establishment," *International Journal of Health Services* (1989); "Radiogenic breast cancer. Effects of mammographic screening," *Journal of the National Cancer Institute* (1986).

CHAPTER 7
STRATEGIES IN CONVENTIONAL MEDICINE

1. George Crile, Jr., *The Way It Was—Sex, Surgery, Treasure and Travel 1907–1987* (Kent, Ohio: Kent State University Press, 1992).
2. Ibid.
3. B. Fisher and C. Redmond, *Studies of the National Surgical Adjuvant Project* (Amsterdam: Elsevier/North-Holland: Biomedical Press, 1977), 67–81.
4. Source obtained from the Internet: www.uhealthnet.on.ca/libraryarchives.htm.
5. Fisher, *Studies of the National Surgical Adjuvant Project,* 67–81.
6. Anonymous, "The chemo's Berlin wall crumbles," *Cancer Chronicles* (December 1990): 4.
7. Ibid.
8. *The Journal of Clinical Oncology* (November 1987).
9. Anonymous, "The chemo's Berlin wall crumbles," *Cancer Chronicles* (December 1990): 4.

10. Ibid.
11. Marion Morra and Eve Potts, *Realistic Alternatives in Cancer Treatment* (New York: Avon Books, 1980), 176.
12. Ibid.
13. George Crile, *Cancer and Common Sense* (New York: Viking Press, 1955).

CHAPTER 8
VICTORY STRATEGIES THROUGH ALTERNATIVE MEDICINE

1. "New Ways of Healing," *MPLS St. Paul* (1994).
2. Internet: www.worldwithoutcancer.com/ hunza.html.
3. Ibid.
4. Ibid.
5. Source obtained from Internet: www.encyclopedia.com/ articles/13588.html.
6. Internet: babelfish.altavista.com/ cgi-bin/translate?
7. Source obtained from Internet: Otto Warburg, "The Prime Cause and Prevention of Cancer," 222.o3zone.com/ ozoneser/articles/034.htm.
8. Wade Roush, "Herbert Benson: Mind-Body maverick pushes the envelope," *Science* 276 (18 April 1997): 357–359.
9. Source obtained from Internet: Renee Twombly, "Use of prayer or noetic therapy may contribute to better outcomes in cardiac patients," www.dukenews.duke.edu/med/ MANTRA2.HTM.
10. Source obtained from Internet: www.csmonitor.com/ durable/1997/09/15/us/us.6.htm.

CHAPTER 9
AN OASIS OF HOPE

1. American Cancer Society, *Cancer Facts and Figures.*
2. Harrison's Principles of Internal Medicine, 9th edition, 1263–1264.
3. American Cancer Society, *Cancer Facts and Figures.*

4. W. A. Sakr et. al., "High grade prostatic intraepithelial neoplasia and prostatic adenocarcinoma between the ages of 20–69: an autopsy study of 249 cases," *In Vivo* 8 (1994):439–443 (obtained from the Internet: www.prostateforum.com/sample.htm).
5. Internet: www.cancer.med.upenn.edu/specialty/surg_onc/ ahcpr_radpc.html; and external.aomc.org/prostate.html.
6. American Cancer Society, *Cancer Facts and Figures.*
7. Ibid.
8. Francois, Duc de La Rochefoucauld, 15th century.

CHAPTER 10
THE POWER OF PREVENTION

1. *Mainichi Daily News,* August 25,1999.
2. Anonymous, "Wasted Health Care Dollars," *Consumer Reports* (July 1992): 435–445.
3. Thomas J. Moore, *Deadly Medicine* (New York: Simon & Schuster, 1995), 121, 219.
4. Harrison's *Principles of Internal Medicine,* 9th edition, 1263–1264.
5. T. Colin Campbell and Christine Cox, *The China Project* (Ithaca, NY: New Century Nutrition, 1996), 16.
6. Select Committee on Nutrition and Human Needs, United States Senate, *Dietary Goals for the United States* (Washington, 1977), 3.
7. Ibid., v.
8. Ibid.
9. Ibid.
10. Ibid.
11. Ibid.
12. *Healthy People: The Surgeon General's Report on Health Promotion and Disease Prevention* (1979); *Promoting Health/Preventing Disease: Objectives for the Nation* (1980).
13. U.S. Department of Health and Human Services, *Dietary Guidelines for Americans,* 1985.

Notes

14. U.S. Department of Health and Human Services, *The Surgeon General's Report on Nutrition and Health,* 1989.
15. Ibid.
16. Ibid.
17. Ibid.
18. Ibid.
19. Internet: www.obesity.org/ what.htm.

CHAPTER 12
GOD'S HEALING WAYS

1. Larry Dossey, *Healing Words* (New York: Harper-Paperbacks, 1957), 250.
2. Ibid.
3. William G. Braud, "Human Interconnectedness: Research Indications," *ReVision* 14, no. 3 (Winter 1992): 140–148.
4. Patch Adams, *House Calls* (San Francisco: Robert D. Reed Publishers, 1998), 124.

CHAPTER 13
RESTORING THE POWER OF HOPE

1. Internet source: touchstarpro.com/siegel.html.

APPENDIX A

1. American Cancer Society, *Cancer Facts and Figures,* 9.

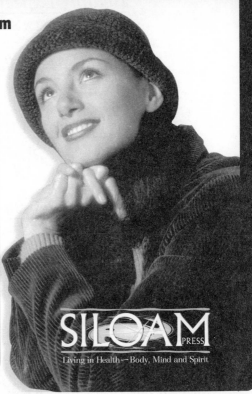

Pick up these other health-related books from Siloam Press:

Walking in Divine Health
BY DON COLBERT, M.D.

The Bible Cure Booklets
BY DON COLBERT, M.D.

You Are Not What You Weigh
BY LISA BEVERE

The Bible Cure
BY REGINALD CHERRY, M.D.

Healthy Expectations
BY PAMELA SMITH

Fit for Excellence!
BY SHERI ROSE SHEPHERD

Ultimate Living!
BY DEE SIMMONS

Train Up Your Children in the Way They Should Eat
BY SHARON BROER

Maximum Energy
BY TED BROER

Available at your local bookstore
or call 1-800-599-5750
or visit our Web site at www.creationhouse.com